AS ALL WOUNDS

AS ALL WOUNDS

VICTOR REARDON

As All Wounds
By Victor Reardon.

Dedications

To Ian, for always looking out for me, and for keeping me motivated and inspired.

To Chuck and Antony, you've saved my life more than you'll ever know—I love you both.

To Tammy and Yasmin, for helping me bring this together.

Acknowledgments

Writing this book has been a long process. A year ago, it seemed almost impossible, but I had a choice: I could either drink myself to death, consumed by depression and shame, or I could pull myself up and give it everything I had. The first step was accepting a few harsh truths.

This is where the book begins—accepting loneliness. I had to face the fact that no one was coming to save me or pull me out of the darkness I had fallen into. In my darkest moments, lying piss-drunk on the floor of my flat, unable to stand or even compose myself—let alone write anything comprehensible—all I wanted to do was die.

But I couldn't.

Every time I closed my eyes, I saw my sister and my nieces. They're growing up so quickly, and the thought of leaving them behind was unbearable. I couldn't stand the idea of the pain my selfish actions would cause my mum.

I would close my eyes and see her too—the life we had, the life I had to accept was gone. The memories of a future we would never have together haunted me.

The thought that the only thing keeping me alive was the hurt my leaving would cause—and realizing it would make no difference to those I love—was overwhelming.

One of the hardest things I've ever had to do followed: accepting the past. There are things I've done in my life that I'll never find peace or acceptance from—the hurt I've caused. I had to bury it and let it go.

Accepting that the past is the past that we can't change it or undo the hurt or pain left behind, is freeing. But we do have a choice in what we do with it. We can let it break us, or we can use it—channel it into something better.

This book is a tribute to that: to accepting loss, grief, and a future I never thought I deserved. This book was born of loss and pain, but it's also about hope. In life's darkest moments, it's okay to hope. I found hope in God, in my friends and family. In those dark times, hope may seem impossible, but I promise you it's not.

The last lesson I learned was this: this too shall pass. Whether it's grief, loss, or happiness, these moments will pass by in the blink of an eye, faster than you can imagine.

I'm nearly thirty now, and I'm not where I thought I would be. I thought I'd be married with kids by now, creating the family I couldn't imagine as a child. But I'm not—and that's okay. We all move at our own pace. If it doesn't happen for me, that's okay too. I've experienced love—amazing, beautiful love—and no matter what happens for the rest of my life, I'll always have that.

I won't lie and tell you that everything is perfect or that all my issues have resolved themselves. I'm still alone. Even in a room full of people, that feeling has never left. But I will tell you this: it's okay not to be okay. Just because things aren't fine now doesn't mean they won't be.

I have faith that everything will work out as it's supposed to. I pray and hope that you do too—that you find the strength to get through whatever comes your way and fight through the darkness. There is light at the end of the tunnel; you just have to keep going, no matter what.

Thank you for taking the time to read this book. It means a lot to me. And if you've read this, reach out to a friend or a loved one. See how they're doing—they might need it.

Dad, I'm sorry I wasn't there for you like you were for me.

I'm sorry things ended the way they did. We were too similar, and we always thought we had more time.

For now, I'll try to make you proud. That's all I ever wanted to do. I'm sorry I never showed you that side of me. Rest peacefully. I'll do my best to look out for Eddie and the girls.

CHAPTER 1

"When you are born in a burning house, you think the world is on fire. But it's not."

- Unknown -

My earliest memory: I'm four years old, staring down the hallway of the house I grew up in. My mum is screaming at my dad to stop arguing with my brother, but it's too late—it has already gone too far.

You know those moments when the adrenaline has peaked, and it's too late for either party to back down?

My father too prideful.

My brother never the type to back down from a fight. It's something I know, in his later years, he would reflect on—something that would haunt him more than he would care to admit.

The thing about violence is that when it's over—when the dust settles and the screaming stops, when you come out on the other side—it's hard not to look back at the path paved with blood that led you there.

I don't know what started this particular conflict. Maybe it was the cheap scotch Dad would sneak behind bath panels and under furniture. The smell would emanate throughout the house once he'd started drinking, coupled with my brother's brash attitude, like a slow-burning fuse. Eventually, the inevitable would happen.

Sometimes, I miss that old house—the funny green wallpaper you'd never pick in a million years, the old TV with the huge back panel where my brother and I would play video games for hours. I think of the time we spent split-screening *James Bond*, an escape from the outside world.

I think he knew what he was doing. When Dad had been drinking, my brother would keep me distracted enough that I wouldn't hear the sirens or the shouting from downstairs. But there's only so much you can cover.

So here we are: I'm standing in that dark hallway, lit only by a single bulb hanging overhead. Mum is screaming again—something I'll never understand to this day. It's never fixed a situation.

Dad's voice used to echo through this house when he was mad. I swear it could have ripped the paint off the walls.

I'll never forget this moment for as long as I live. Dad's screaming—I'm so young I don't even know what about. The dim lighting highlights the fear on my brother's face. He doesn't know what to do; he's so young. To this day, I remember every detail of his face—fresh, smooth. He hadn't been scarred by life yet.

Dad's screaming now, so loud that Mum is worrying about the neighbours. Funny, right? He's turning red with alcoholic rage, on the verge of destroying everyone in this house, and she's worried the neighbours might be a little miffed. Thanks, Mum.

It's the little details that stick with you: that dimly lit bulb, the smell of scotch and stale roll-ups—so strong that even now, saying this, forty years on, it still makes me queasy. And I'm not a soft man, nor is my disposition anything less than stellar.

I know this moment stuck with you too, bro, and I'm sorry I couldn't stop it. I'm so fucking sorry because you'll never know this, but I didn't forget! Trust me, I didn't forget. When the time came, you best believe I gave that man fucking hell for you!

Ten years later, he tried the same shit with me. He pushed me so hard, I still remember the sound of my head hitting the wall behind me. I felt the warmth of my blood almost instantly. And the look on his face when I buried my fist in it would have made you so proud. I mean, he kicked the absolute shit out of me for it, but you best believe I went down swinging. For the first time in my life, I saw that man could be hurt.

I stood helplessly at the end of the hallway, watching you and him sparring back and forth, verbally tearing into each other. Something snapped. You never told me what was said, but the fear in your face when he grabbed you haunted me for a long time. In a way, it still does.

I was always so proud of you. Even in the face of unavoidable danger, you never backed down. You never stopped giving everything you had to protect me. I know you always put me before yourself.

When he grabbed you, your entire demeanor shifted into something nasty. Don't misunderstand me when I say this—growing up, nasty is how you survive. It's how *we* survived.

It wouldn't be until many years later that you would face a similar situation at a house party. We were both selling water in pipettes, passing them off as drug enhancers to tripped-out dickheads, when some young kid with a reputation for being hot-headed thought it would be funny to try robbing you in front of his pals.

I've never seen someone get back up as fast as they hit the ground, and I know he didn't expect you to throw a head-butt so hard that you sprayed his friends with his blood. Growing up, this was how we made it home.

And when Dad grabbed you, I know your life changed. The noise he made when he hit you for the first time sounded like thunder. How you managed to stay upright, I'll never figure out, but I remember the first punch you threw back before he grabbed you by the neck, digging his nails in while he did. That's the thing about Dad—he didn't just want to beat you. He wanted to hurt you. He wanted you to look back at the scars he left. He wanted you to know what he was capable of.

I know you gave it everything you could, and I think that's why it hurts more—because it didn't change anything. It didn't stop him from leaving your blood pooling at the bottom of the wash hamper he used to hold you against while hitting you with the other hand.

And life isn't a movie. You don't take all those punches and walk away. I know you were unconscious by the second or third, and by the sixth, Mum tried pulling him off you.

I'll never blame you, you know, for leaving—Eddie too. Sometimes the pain becomes too unbearable, and we don't see a way out. I just wish you knew how much you meant to me. You were never asked to protect me, but you did it every single day without a second thought, without hesitation, and with a tenacity that very few people could match.

The thing is—that's my first memory.

They didn't get better after that.

And I couldn't adjust. This is the thing about violence—at the moment, you're fine. Better than fine. Fucking alive. But when the dust settles, and all that's left is swollen knuckles and guilt, it's hard not to look back with remorse and wonder if things could have been different. But you taught me—that's not possible.

When we lost Harry, I know he didn't want that fight. He tried everything to avoid it, but it didn't mean fuck all—he was dead before he hit the ground. I think after that, we understood. Losing Harry taught us that sometimes you've got to fight back. Losing you taught me there's a time to walk away.

My first love was called Hannah. She was one of those rare people whose beauty on the inside could only be rivaled by her beauty on the outside. She had brown eyes that I could read from anywhere in the room and long hair that often fell in front of her face—something that melted my heart every single time. She had a smile that could light the darkest room.

The way she looked at me brought a peace to my soul I never thought possible. I couldn't figure it out. Sometimes, when the world fell apart, when the sky seemed to be falling and all hope was lost, she would wrap her hands around my arm, and just like that, everything would be okay.

What did she see in me?

I didn't deserve her from the start.

But she stayed, despite everything—despite all the violence, all the horror. She was the first person to ever look at me like I wasn't fucking broken.

Which made it all the harder when she left.

She was an angel—softly spoken but headstrong. She was someone who knew what she wanted and didn't let anyone or anything stop her from getting there. But she was naive to the world and how it works.

When she started hanging around with Sam, I told her what he was like.

"He's like a brother to me," she would say.

"He's not like other guys."

Please don't think for a second that I'm ever going to put an ounce of blame on Hannah's name. We were both too young and stupid for this world.

That day, I just had a bad feeling. As much as it annoyed me, I would never have asked her not to hang out with him or anyone else.

Your happiness is all that matters.

I would have cut out my own heart to prove that to you.

I think, in a way, I did.

Rushing home, I prayed that you were okay. I called and called, and when you didn't answer, panic set in.

I've never been fazed by much, but the thought of you hurting—words can't describe it.

I almost took the door off its hinges coming through it, seeing the fear on your face as you kicked at him, desperately trying to keep him away. And for what happened next, I know we both wished we could change it.

I pulled him off you and tripped him over his jeans, which he had pulled down to his knees while trying to hurt you. Then, I took my foot and aimed it straight for his temple.

And I'm sorry for two things. I'm sorry he tried to hurt you, and I'm sorry you had to witness that side of me—a side I tried to kill.

You never looked at me the same after that. I get it, and I don't blame you at all. Of course, it hurts. Every single day it hurts. But I understand. And at the end of all this, your happiness is all that matters, whether I'm in your life or not.

I knew I had to leave after that. But I'll tell you this: I'd kill him again. I'd kill him a thousand times if it meant your safety, if it meant you got to stay yourself. I wouldn't think twice.

So here we are. And I feel like if you've found these letters, then you already know what I've done. It means things didn't work out for me. So first, I should apologize.

To Eddie: I wasn't the best brother. We both know it. The truth is, being around you was too hard. It wasn't fair to you. Let's be honest—me being around you was just a reminder of how fucking awful things used to be. And you've got the girls now. They don't need me in their lives. They don't need to explain to their friends who the old man with the scarred knuckles is, or reassure them that he's friendly when they just want to run a mile.

And to be honest, the only reason I lasted as long as I have is because of you—because I thought you needed me. The last time I saw you, I came home. I didn't say anything; I wanted to surprise you. And I caught you, just for a moment. You chased the girls inside. I could hear their giggles. I saw you—happy. I mean, truly happy.

That was enough for me. You made it. I couldn't ask for anything else.

But while we're here, I should say a few things.

First, about money. There's about fifty grand in savings for you. It's not much, but I never had kids, never really spent much. Sell everything else. Use it to look after the girls.

Make sure they're looked after first.

I never had kids; I was so scared of ending up like Dad that the thought never fully processed in my head. Maybe in another life.

Know that I'm at peace. Don't cry for me—I'm okay, I really am. This isn't something I've done on a whim. I've thought about it.

I had love. I had an amazing love that was pure and beautiful, if brief, and I shall take that with me.

Check in with Hannah and tell her there's nothing either of us could have done. Sometimes, that's life.

Yeah, it sucks, and it hurts every day, but I'd take that pain every single time if it meant she didn't have to. Just look after her. I don't want her blaming herself. This is on me. I was too weak to shoulder this life anymore.

Lastly, remember me as a good man—not this useless shell that's been left, but a good man. That's all I ever wanted to be, really.

I had this thought, lying with Hannah one morning. She was snoring loud enough that cars passing by sped up to avoid what they probably thought was an earthquake. I laid there, watching her sleep—at peace, real peace.

There's something I used to ask you every day: *Do you feel loved? Do you feel safe and protected?*

I always wondered if you understood why I asked that, but I never explained, and I'm grateful you never pressed me to. I think you knew me well enough to put two and two together.

So, I'm watching her sleep, listening to that deep snore—one that could have scared off a bear—but honestly, I thought it was adorable. And I imagined what our life would be.

I never thought I'd have kids. But with her, I saw it. I saw us having a child, maybe two; raising them, teaching them right from wrong. I imagined days at the zoo, showing them all the wonderful things this life has to offer.

I saw us growing old together, looking back on the years of wonder we built—the home we created, the family we raised. A home where they felt safe, where we laughed. A kitchen where we argued, and a bedroom where we made up.

I think one of the hardest parts of losing her was losing the life we were supposed to have together. I've felt like I've been mourning another life—one that, in an instant, was ripped away from us.

I do wonder if she thinks about me. Does she ever wonder how I'm doing? What I'm up to? Like I do her.

I don't know if she's moved on. I was too scared to reach out.

The thought of you with another man—laughing, holding him—would you hold his arm the way you used to hold mine? Or take his hand when you get excited? The thought is paralyzing. In one breath, all I want is your happiness, whether that's with me or not. But in the other, I know in my heart it should have been with me.

So, I'll leave you to it. I'll leave you alone because I can't stay—it'll hurt too much. But I hope you find the happiness I couldn't give you.

If I'm going to do this, then I'm going to do it right—or as right as one can in this particular situation. I'm going to Wakefield, for a couple of reasons really. In years past, this is where my grandparents met.

As Grandma tells it, she looked at Grandad across the hall of a little club known as *Little India*. She took one look at him, turned to her friends, and said, "I'm going to marry that man." And that she did.

Seventy blissful years they had together before she passed. I remember asking Grandad how a love like that could exist and what it felt like. He looked at me, took my hand, and just said, "If I could relive my life again, I wouldn't change a single moment... because I got to meet her." That's the kind of love most people will never find in their lives.

We are born into this world alone and afraid, and we spend our lives following the slow march of time as we grow, learning from those who came before us.

My mother used to tell me, "Something worth doing is worth doing well," or "If you're bored, you're boring." And my favorite—she'd say it anytime she started an ice-cold cola or felt the sun beaming down on her face, "It's the little things in life," she'd tell me with a little smile.

This is why I like Wakefield. There's something about the people here; it's a different world. When I left the army, I would come down here on a hot summer day, drink a Whitfield's, a popular local Irish beer that was silky smooth. Something about the Gladiator on the bottle always made me chuckle. And I would just watch the world go by. Some of the most beautiful people on the planet live here—they really do.

The last time I was here, I met a fighter. Isla was her name. We sat and had a beer, and she told me about her dad and how he had raised her boxing. But he opposed violence; he would always tell her to leave first, that her pride wasn't worth the fall. He taught her how to fight so she would never have to.

I wish he'd met my dad, you know.

CHAPTER 2

We grow, not by years,
But tears and heartbreaks
- Rithvik Singh -

It's midnight, and the train to Wakefield barrels along quietly under the cover of the night sky. I must have worn these old shoes down to the skin with how many times I've wandered these carriages. Since serving, something about public transport makes me uneasy.

You know, sometimes you come under gunfire, and your heartbeat doesn't change at all. I remember feeling the shattering of hot embers bouncing off a wall behind me, caused by shrapnel. At that moment, I remember just feeling numb... ready.

But on my last tour, I was sent to a local village to check on the residents—nothing suspicious, just routine in and out, checking on the people, enjoying the scenery, and light work.

I sat in the back of our pickup truck, watching the early sunrise over the village. The orange sky slowly took over the farmlands, morning mist covering what the sun didn't, and the smell of fresh wheat fields crawling through our cab.

But something felt off; something felt wrong. In my heart, I couldn't figure it out, but I sat up quicker than the hairs on my neck could react. Coming through the morning smog, the first thing I noticed was the relative normality of the place. I can't put my finger on it, but something about the lack of anything being off threw me.

We parked our truck on the side of town and took a slow walk through, always stopping to chat with locals—often using this as an opportunity to learn the land and get to better understand local cultures and customs.

The thing about this particular deployment is that we were never meant to see action; our mission was to observe and report. Why they even bothered to issue us firearms was beyond me. Our entire purpose for being here was just to help bridge the gap between a new regime and old customs.

I put the safety on my rifle and slung it over my back, lit a cigarette, and made my way slowly through town, stopping to chat with an old couple. They told me about the lighthouse on the hill—St. Brandon, it was called. The legend was that a single man, Brandon, held off a militia once, using the narrow stairway of the lighthouse and whatever supplies he could find until the local cavalry could come for aid.

I loved stories like that—not just the lone gunman walking into town, but the grit and determination the human body and spirit are capable of under such immense stress. I've seen men and women discover parts of themselves under fire that they never thought themselves capable of.

And the one thing I could tell you above anything about St. Brandon, the protector of the lighthouse and savior of this small village, is that not only was he a warrior, but he was also a good man.

"Excuse me, sir," a man called out, shuffling slowly towards me. I walked towards him, keeping hold of the rifle strap to make sure it didn't leave my back. They were hard-working, good people, and the last thing they needed was us causing fear in their village.

He explained that our presence here had caused a ripple in the community. He knew we meant no harm, but not everyone did. They saw rifles and, rightfully so, made assumptions; some had packed up and left, while others began barricading their homes.

"Here's the thing, though—Tony, my neighbor—he boarded his windows up days ago, and no one's seen or heard from them since. He's got kids, sir."

Fear does a lot of strange things to a person; it can fell the biggest of men.

So, I followed this man across the town, taking stock of all the windows. Some were filled with eyes watching with harsh scrutiny, while others were blocked by wood or shutters. Thinking back on it, for the most part, this town was just like any other: people lived day to day, worked eight hours a day, while their kids went to school.

But then, sometimes, the town would be riddled with bullets and gunpowder smoke. It's fascinating, really, the resolve of these great people to remain unfazed by all that their government had failed to stop.

Coming up to the neighbor's house, even now, after all these years, I think back on it. If I could tell myself, I wouldn't have gone into that fucking house. There was nothing amiss, really; thinking back on it, the windows were a little dirty, but nothing I would have thought to investigate. I crept slowly up the front steps before knocking loudly to announce my presence.

Nothing.

I unholstered my pistol, and holding onto the door handle with my right hand, I forced the door open, breaking the locks as I did. As that door opened, I knew exactly what had happened. As the light hit the inside door and fresh air hit the moist, dusty interior, immediate dread filled my throat. The smell of rotten flesh mixed with an almost sweet undertone filled the air, hitting every sense along the way.

The first room—the living room—was clear; nothing was touched. The kitchen still had dirty dishes in the sink. We've all done it: "I'll get them in the morning." Something told me I should turn around when my foot hit the first step. That smell seemed to double in strength with every step. It wasn't long before the old boy had turned around and made his way back out into the fresh air. I could hear him vomiting outside from the top of the stairs.

As much as I wished I could have done the same, something told me I needed to keep going. I holstered my weapon; I knew it was too late. I decided to follow the smell and rip off that Band-Aid. Whatever I was going to find was not going to be good.

I followed the smell to the first room past the stairs and pushed it open slowly. The sound of flies buzzing was so loud I could feel the vibrations through my feet. What lay before me, I don't think I'll ever forget for the rest of my life.

Two beds separated by only a few feet: the left had a child lying still, one gunshot to her head—she didn't even wake up. The second bed—I assumed the child had heard the gunshot and tried to run in panic—she didn't make it: one shot to the back of the head.

Tony, panicked by what he thought would be an unstoppable war, had spent most of the evening making his way through a bottle of Handsome Jack's, an old whiskey, smooth and expensive. He then took himself upstairs and shot his child asleep in her bed, the other in the back when she tried to run out of the house.

He then took himself into his room, shot his wife, and lay down beside her, putting the barrel in his mouth and shooting himself. I've done a lot of bad things in my life. I've hurt more people than I care to think about; I've broken people, broken hearts, and faced demons I hope most never have to endure. A lot of this comes down to survival.

Sometimes you have no choice. It's important to distinguish those moments, but this man...Tony, I'll see him in hell.

As the train barreled through on its way to Wakefield, between bouts of whiskey and cheeky cigarettes out of the train window, I was taken back to my first date with Hannah. There was something about her eyes; there was a way she looked at me that has stuck with me. I'll never meet anyone as long as I live who looked at me the way she did. It was like she could see into my soul; she knew me better than I knew myself.

Sometimes we would be out in a crowd full of people, and I always told her it was only her I saw. She had this way of containing her excitement when the food arrived at a restaurant, or I would always know where she would be sitting in a coffee shop; I'd look for the pushchairs or the dogs on leashes.

I've never been good in crowds. Hannah knew this about me; she could tell. I don't know if it was due to me being vertically challenged or my time in the army, but I've always been on edge in crowds. She would hold my forearm tight, and every time, I knew things would be okay.

The day I knew we were over...that look changed. I wish I could put it into words, but it's like she was looking at someone else. I'll never forget that—the day my heart split and was never pieced together.

"Another whiskey, sir?" The smiling cart attendant asked, the bags under her eyes weighing her down. I just nodded.

"What's your name?"

"Tim... and yourself?"

"Steph. I'm sorry, Tim, you aren't meant to smoke here."

"I'm sorry; I'm putting it out."

"Wait," she said, moving to shut the carriage door, looking both ways down the aisle before she did, and walking back in. She took the cigarette from Tim, slumping herself down in the seat opposite him and taking a long drag—a long, peaceful drag.

"Long day?"

For the next hour, Tim and Steph swapped stories between smoke and whiskey. A Wakefield-born-and-bred resident, she lived in her old family home alone. It turned out her father was a soldier who had passed during his last tour. She had always thought about selling the house and jumping on this train heading out of Wakefield, but as with most people who come here, they don't want to leave.

I get that.

Steph was young—late twenties—but her eyes told a tale as old as time, that of pain and hardship. She knew the struggles of seeing her dad return home and readjusting to... civilian problems, you could call it. It is a strange transition that seems alien from the outside. We live every day with the acceptance of the inevitable, and not everyone comes home, but being bonded in blood and hellfire to coming home to parking tickets and people complaining about their coffee orders being wrong.

That is always the one that got me. I stood behind an older, portly lady in a coffee shop screaming at the poor barista in front of her that her non-soy, sugar-free, whipped bullshit was wrong, and I remember thinking to myself, "This is the freedom I fought for? I'd take gunfire any day."

"Thank you. A lot of people come through here, you know? You're the first that's ever asked my name," Steph said, taking a final drag, throwing the lit butt out the window, and closing her eyes... slowly drifting off.

I took my coat off her and placed it gently over her.

As the train rolled in, Tim pulled his coat up over Steph, making sure not to wake her, before grabbing a single bag from the overhead and making his way into the town. The sun was slowly rising over Wakefield, leaving a mesmerizing orange hue that filled the sky. He stopped and closed his eyes, feeling the cold air wash over him.

He had never thought about it before, but if this was to be one of the last sunrises he would ever see, he was going to soak up every ounce of it he could.

CHAPTER 3

This too shall pass
         – Unknown –

It had been more than twenty-four hours since Tim had slept, and with whiskey still flowing through his bloodstream, he wandered through the town, stopping by all the places he and Hannah had visited. The coffee shop featured a giant David Bowie mural that no one could explain, while food trucks opened with the rising sun. They had tried every single one, fueled by the sheer excitement of the hustle and bustle, inhaling the smell of pulled beef and cumin in the air, along with the aroma of freshly fried chips.

Wakefield slumbered, but when it awoke, it did so with a fierce energy, bursting into life.

Tim staggered past the now bustling food fans, navigating through the waking town as he made his way down to the beach. Wakefield was famous for its stunning beaches, with beautiful blue seas and silky-smooth sand. The chilly morning air swept over the water, sending fresh breezes toward Tim. The cold air hit him like a punch, causing him to stumble backward, his backside knocking sand into his pockets.

Tim reached into his pockets and dusted off the now crumpled cigarette packet. He took the last smoke from it, reached back into the same pocket, and pulled out a little black book. After taking a single drag, he began to write.

"Hey, Hannah,

If you've got this, it means things didn't work out for me. I'll keep this short. Firstly, I want to say I'm sorry. I'm sorry things didn't work out; I'm sorry you had to see that side of me.

I know I wasn't always the easiest person to deal with. I can't stop thinking about the day we met. I'll never forget seeing you coming up those stairs with your double-strapped backpack and a cheeky grin. Your smile was the first thing I saw, and to this day, there hasn't been a sunrise or a view on this planet that could match that beauty.

Since the day we met, you have been my every thought—my first thought when waking up and my last thought before I went to sleep. I still have a photo of the day we met. Funny, right? How many people do you reckon can say that?

I hope you meet someone who can give you what I never could. Do me one thing, though, please! Remember me as a good man. That's all I ever wanted to be. With you, I finally felt like I had a chance to be just that; maybe I had a chance to be the man my dad wasn't, to have the family I never had, and with you gone, that dream died.

Your leaving was the hardest thing I've ever experienced in my life, and second to that was mourning the life we never got to have. You are and always have been my everything—my heart until the last beat.

Goodbye, Han.

Tim"

CHAPTER 4

Tim pulled himself up and stumbled across the beach, putting the letter into the nearest post box he could find before stumbling back to the beach, taking a final pull on his cigarette, closing his eyes, and passing out...

"Tim, wake the fuck up."

"Dad?"

"I said get the fuck up," Steve said, grabbing young Tim by the legs and pulling him out of bed. His head hit the laminated flooring as he fell.

The smell of stale cider and day-old cigarette smoke lingered in the room; this would burn your eyes if you came unprepared—another night, another bout.

Tim pulled himself to his feet and wiped the blood from his eye. He looked his dad up and down, noticing the wobble in his stance and how he tried to maintain his balance despite alcohol winning this particular battle.

Tim had watched his dad stagger about, knocking books off the shelf and desperately trying to maintain some sense of self. Between bouts of screaming and missed punches, he looked around at the now trashed room. He never placed much stock in material items but valued the pride in maintaining his personal space—something that would carry through into his army days.

He took one step forward, and with every ounce of power he could muster, Tim swung at his dad, knocking him clear off his feet and sending him hurtling backward, smashing through the units of books and DVDs and knocking them onto the floor.

Steve's eyes rolled back into his skull, and he was gone to the world.

Tim watched his dad lie unconscious on the floor and looked around the room for something. He hadn't figured it out yet, but he knew he'd recognize it when he saw it. Before walking over to his bed and grabbing a pillow, he walked slowly back to his dad, placing a knee on either side of his snoozing body. He then dropped down and forced the pillow into his dad's face, using all his weight to hold him down.

Within seconds, he felt his dad's hands reach up, battling to regain his breath. The longer Tim held him down, the more desperate he became, kicking his legs and screaming, the sounds muffled through the pillow. He quickly realized that no one was coming.

Tim felt a rush of adrenaline pulse through him. "This is it! This is the fucking moment! For everything you've ever done, you sick fuck!" Tim thought to himself.

Tim pulled the pillow off his dad and could see the fear in his eyes. He lay there in shock, not saying a word.

"Fuck you!" he screamed. Steve still hadn't moved; he was a bully, plain and simple. There had been very few times in his life when anyone had ever really stood up to him. He had gotten through life like this, screaming and shouting into the wind and never expecting anything to come back.

"I need to get out of this house," Tim said to himself, trying to regain control of his breath. He pulled himself up and made his way out of his room, across the landing. As he got close to the stairs, he felt a razor-sharp slash to his back that sent him flying down the stairs before he lost consciousness. His last memory was the warm feeling of blood rolling down his forehead, covering his eyes. He could see Steve coming down the stairs, his eyes not leaving Tim's.

"Fuck you," Steve whispered, gently pulling off his belt.

CHAPTER 5

We must be willing to let go of the life we planned to have the life that is waiting for us.

– Joseph Campbell –

"Excuse me, sir."

"Sir, are you alive?"

Tim awoke to the sounds of waves crashing and cold air shooting through his body. As he pulled himself up, his head began to crash like the waves of water in front of him. The young voice that had woken him had gone, scurrying across the beach in fear—maybe it was the bloodshot eyes or the smell of day-old whiskey that lingered on his person.

He stumbled to his feet and took a long, deep breath, feeling the cold air on his face and enjoying this moment; despite everything, in this moment, there was nothing to fear.

Walking back through the town, Tim stopped to grab a newspaper and a fresh pack of cigarettes. He stopped in a coffee shop and sat outside, watching the world go by: the hustle of the street vendors working every angle to try and make a living. He saw the kids playing in the street, racing their bikes and causing the usual tomfoolery that kids do.

The thing that struck him the most, though, was a young couple, both beautiful. He was taken aback by the happiness they exuded as the young man pushed a small pram, his part-ner's purse slung over his shoulder. It was obvious from the outset that this young gentleman was doing everything he could to ease the pain of his partner after childbirth. He wasn't taking any chances, even angling the pram so he could pull open the door of the coffee shop for this beautiful young lady.

"Our kids would be amazing, you know," Hannah said, ly-ing next to Tim, running her long nails through his hair and looking deeply into his eyes.

"Well, of course, if they had your looks and brains... and overall personality, and my..." Tim chuckled.

"You are a good man, Tim! A great man! If our kids were half as patient and kind as you are, I think we're going to be okay."

Making his way to the little hotel that sat overlooking the beach, Tim admired the wooden porch that swung around the front—not something you saw a lot of around here, but he loved the Southern American vibe it gave off.

He had always thought about having a proper home him-self—that's something he would have liked: BBQs out back, beers on the front deck watching the sun go down with Han-nah as they traded stories and swapped songs, something they'd done since their first date.

The hotel kept the same aesthetic on the inside, like walk-ing into an old saloon in a western; the hotel reception even bore a similar resemblance to an old bar.

"Maybe a duel at high noon if I'm lucky," he chuckled to himself.

"Can I help you, sir?" a voice called out.

"Tim, I booked a room. Genuine question... is this place... western-themed?"

"No," she said sternly.

"That'll be a deposit of £199." Tim reached into his pockets to find his card, and it became apparent very quickly...

"The kid!" he said.

"One moment."

"Three doors down," the receptionist chuckled. "That's Luke, little rascal. Don't be too hard on him, will you?"

Leaving his bag, Tim made his way out and down the road before coming to the house the lady had told him about through held-back laughter.

Tim had found the house but couldn't quite understand why she had asked him not to go hard on the young lad. "Best believe I'm going to give him the discipline his parents haven't," he thought to himself. Walking up the driveway, he couldn't help but judge, seeing the overgrown weeds growing through the patio and the unkempt pathway. These weren't people who took pride in their household—another thought he should probably keep to himself—before banging loudly on the front door.

Instantly, the door swung open, and there stood Luke, fear in his eyes and tears streaming down his face.

"Help me!" he pleaded, turning and running back upstairs.

Following up the stairs, Tim couldn't help but scan the house. It wasn't messy by any means but was dirty, with dust covering every unit, windows glazed, and bugs dead on the seals.

As Tim rounded the corner, he could see the young boy had already sprung into action. He had rolled his dad into a side position, his right hand grabbing a knee and his left hand clutching his shoulder.

Tim rushed behind and applied three hard slaps to his dad's back, dislodging whatever it was he had ingested that had caused his breathing to stop. The blueness in his face slowly returned to a pale white, and the old boy patted Tim gently on the hand.

"Thanks, son," he said, taking a breath, closing his eyes, and drifting off.

"Thank you!" Luke said, handing Tim back his debit card with a look of guilt and appreciation. He had recognized Tim almost immediately, but in his desperate attempt to get help, he knew this was something he had to put to bed, if only temporarily.

"Please stay for dinner," Luke asked. The young lad stood no more than four feet tall, with ragged red hair and bright green eyes. It became very apparent quickly that this was his life—not one he had asked for, but one he had accepted. There was a defiance and toughness in him that Tim had seen only in his brothers in arms.

He politely declined and took himself back to the hotel.

CHAPTER 6

Dear Eddie,

I've got some explaining to do, firstly this isn't on you. This is on me, I'm sorry I haven't been around much, the truth is being around you hurts.

It hurts being the reminder of how fucked things used to be.

I see the girls in you, they are beautiful, perfect really.

I guess some good can come out of our terrible lives, right?

Make sure you tell them how much I love them!

Know that I'm sorry, this weight got too heavy to carry.

I Love You.

T.

CHAPTER 7

I won't write too many of these, to be honest. There aren't many people who would care. Life moves quickly, and in the mad scramble of our day-to-day routines, it's easy to feel lost.

Tim sat alone on the beach, watching the sun set over the now calm waves, which crashed quietly against the rock faces. Sipping tequila, he needed to plan these final days carefully. Sending the letters was a must; the first one was done—perhaps the most important one.

One last decent meal was essential! A Handsome Jack and a cigarette would be a nice touch; what's a hundred-pound bottle of whiskey to the dead?

Every person you meet knows a different version of you. To one, you may be a hero; to others, a monster. We judge quickly, and every moment after meeting someone is colored by those initial impressions. I once had a meeting with a higher-up who didn't stand to shake any of our hands. Something about that interaction didn't sit right with me, and the rest of the meeting was spent thinking of ways to escape.

When I met Hannah, it was a brief encounter. She had come to inquire about my workplace, and I was besotted. I don't know if it was her smile or the warmth of her presence, but something about her made me obsessed almost instantly. It felt like I had found the missing piece of my soul. I would look for excuses to talk to her whenever she was around, just enough to build up the courage to ask if she would like to go for coffee with me. That scared me more than gunfire.

But she never judged. She knew my childhood; she knew my story, and she stayed—something I didn't think would ever happen in my lifetime.

That day I'll never forget. She had this bright blue cardigan on with two oversized buttons and a silver heart necklace resting neatly on her collarbone. Her long black hair hung over her right shoulder, and the way the sun reflected off her skin amazed me. She had a spotlight wherever she went.

I wish I could have told her how beautiful she was. It was only later that I would find out the beauty on the outside was matched by the beauty on the inside.

My friends would joke, saying, "Honestly, if we didn't know you, we would think you paid her to be with you." They weren't wrong, but beauty is only skin deep.

The moment I knew she was the one, I woke in the night, echoes of a past life battling for control of my sleep. Some nights were harder than others. I woke sweating, breathing heavily, and in a panic. I began counting the blue items I could see around the room—something my psychologist had told me to do as a way of grounding myself when those memories came back.

And without thinking, she placed a hand on my back and one on my arm. Something about the warmth of her touch brought me back to reality. She took my head and rested it against her chest, laying with her legs around me and pulling me down, running her fingers through my hair and speaking calmly.

"It's okay; I've got you," she would say. "You're safe." Like the sweetest symphony, I was back in the room, and the voices and the screaming all stopped.

I would never have asked her to be that person, to shoulder any burden of pain. How could you ask that of someone? But she didn't hesitate, not for a second. For the first time in my entire life, I wasn't alone. I had a home, and I had peace. Sometimes I still wake up in the night, roll over to grab her, and it takes a second before I realize that she isn't there anymore. That's a hurt I will never get used to.

"My dad wants to talk to you," a voice called out, pulling Tim back to reality. He looked around to see Luke standing behind him, hesitant and worried. They both knew he had stolen Tim's card, and Luke was concerned that he would remember and take some kind of revenge. He had never been caught before.

Feeling the tequila coursing through him, Tim debated making the journey over. His head spun slowly as he attempted to drown his sorrows on that lonely beach. Almost tumbling back down, he pulled himself up to his feet and began following the young lad, a little slower than he would have liked, but some battles you have to choose.

"My son says you saved my life. He also says he stole from you."

"It's not a bother, sir. I'm just glad you are okay." Tim scanned the man; there was something about him he recognized—a familiarity he had found with few men on his travels.

"You're a soldier?"

"Marine. Name's Norman." Norman was a short man, slim and frail, but in this state right now, he had something in his eyes—a levity rarely seen in men of this age or in men who had seen combat like these two.

Norman pulled himself up out of bed and made his way across to Tim, making sure to stand at attention and salute, an instinct that seemed to come naturally.

These men had never met before, never exchanged more words than this sentence, but they both knew they were bonded by something deeper than they could explain. Tim stayed for a while; they swapped war stories over the remaining tequila, and Norman explained, "When I got sick, my wife left me. I don't blame her; I don't. Luke has looked after me ever since. He's a good kid, but he hasn't had a childhood—not really, not like he deserves."

That all felt too familiar. Tim knew that feeling instantly; he hadn't had a chance to enjoy his childhood despite his brothers' best efforts. He took a sip of his tequila and looked over at Luke, sleeping peacefully on the ratty sofa across the room.

"I just wanted to say thank you. Whatever you're planning on doing here, the world would be worse off for it."

Tim looked up in shock.

"Don't lie to me, son. I've been there when I fell sick. Trust me, I've been there! But I thank God every single day I didn't listen to any of the fucking dumb thoughts that went through my head!"

Tim tried to scramble together some words and get a better understanding of Norman's words, but nothing came out.

"You can't lie to me, son," he said, taking Tim's hand and squeezing it. "When you are born into a burning house, you think the world is on fire. But it is not. For anyone who's been through trauma, it's very easy to assume everyone is against you."

The first time I took Hannah for dinner, I picked her up flowers on the way—nice ones; they were called Rainbow Joy. I'll never forget them. I got there early, slipped the waiter a little cash to keep us in the front of his mind, and took every opportunity I could to show her that she was the only person in the room I cared about.

She would tell me a little down the line that all the things I did that night—all the little things: opening doors, the flowers, checking in with her, making sure she felt safe and comfortable—were things her ex had done after he had acted up.

It took a lot of patience and understanding before she felt comfortable enough with me doing those sorts of things. I'd have waited a thousand lifetimes if it meant seeing her smile; I guess that's what has made this easier.

It hurts. It does hurt knowing I'll never hold her again or feel her warmth again. I will always look for her smile in any crowd; she is the only person who could stand out in a sea of people by the brightness of her smile.

And I think it hurts more knowing she loves me. I know she still loves me; I can hear it in her voice. The last time we spoke, you told me how much you missed me. I begged you to come home, and you just said, "I can't." You'll always be amazed at how many times your own heart can break.

Tim lay on the floor of his room, his head spinning. He had passed out drunk at some point and hadn't built the motivation or momentum to pull himself up. He just stared at the ceiling, wondering if it would ever stop spinning. He thought of a time when things didn't seem so archaic; closing his eyes, he remembered his Christmas.

"Hey, son, you awake?" his dad had whispered. His dad's smile was the only thing he could see from his tired eyes, the morning grog, his mum would call it, before being led downstairs. Dad was always serious, broken from long workdays and a work ethic that would put a horse to shame, but he was smiling—almost giddy.

"December 27th, 1977. I was your age when my dad showed me, and now I get to show you!" This may have been the last time I was happy. I was five years old, sitting on my dad's lap, watching *Star Wars*! The excitement in his face at getting to introduce me to a pivotal part of his childhood—I remember feeling him watching me, seeing my childlike wonder. He knew every step, every action beat, every laugh.

Dad did a lot of bad things in his life; he hurt a lot of people and pushed more away than I'm sure he cared to think about. But he wasn't always that way. I'll never know what pushed him to become the man he did. It is hard not to think of him as the man who taught me right from wrong, the man who taught me that there is a time to stand up and be counted!

He was a kid when my mum got pregnant—nineteen years old and hadn't even left college yet—but he told me, "I knew what I had to do, and I'd do it again every time." It breaks my heart that this man, the strongest man in the world to me, could be broken by the demons of his mind! I'll never forgive myself for not catching it, for not doing what I know he would have done for me; he would have stopped at nothing.

We'll meet again one day; I know that. I was never a religious man until I met Hannah. Her mere presence gave me a belief that years of bloodshed never could. How could someone so beautiful come to a life like mine? There must be a god. We'll meet again one day, and I hope we can sit down again, like when I was a kid, and maybe he can make some sense of this. He would tell me I'm being a goose; he always knew when I needed sympathy and when he needed to tell me straight.

We'll meet again one day. We'll fight; I promise to God we'll fight! But I hope that we find the peace in death we could never find in life. I'm sorry, Dad.

Tim sat up and reached for the half-empty bottle of whiskey he had dropped when he passed out. The floor around him was scattered with painkillers he had dropped when he hit the ground, one of the few ways he had contemplated taking his own life. He had thought about mixing painkillers with a whiskey chaser, maybe taking a stroll down to the beach and walking out into the sea.

Something about this unsettled him. He knew somebody had to find him—his body. The idea of his bloated corpse being discovered by a random dog walker or school kids didn't sit right with him.

Tim sat on the floor, rolling the pills in his hand like dice, the anxiety in his chest pounding. This is it! This is it! he repeated to himself, slamming another shot.

"Tim," Hannah's voice echoed through his head. "I'll always love you."

"I'll love you too," he whispered to himself, the whiskey burning his throat. His head spun; every time he closed his eyes, that's all he could see—her smile and the warmth it gave, those fucking brown eyes! Tears streamed down his face as his hands shook, bringing them to his mouth.

"I'm sorry, Hannah."

CHAPTER 8

It is during our darkest moments that we must focus to see the light.

– Unknown –

Hands shaking, Tim closed his eyes and took a breath, facing the acceptance of what is, what has been, and what will be. The culmination of years of pain, heartbreak, and violence had weighed on his conscience for too long.

In life, we learn through failure, although by that logic, he often joked to himself that he must be a master in all fields by now.

Then there was a knock at the door.

"Oh, please, not now," he thought to himself, his hands still trembling.

Tim swung open the door to see Luke standing there. The calm look on Luke's face disappeared upon seeing the disheveled appearance of Tim. His eyes were bloodshot, and it didn't take much to see how his tears had burned them. The smell of whiskey and smoke was stronger than Luke had noticed before.

"Dad needs your help," Luke said, worry filling his young face.

Tim turned and grabbed his coat.

"Before we go... please, brush your teeth. You stink," he said.

He followed Luke across the beach and back to the house, swinging open the door to see Norman sitting upright in his chair. He wore a tweed flat cap and a nice grey suit that was a little too tight; it had been a while.

"We thought you might like to go out for dinner."

This wasn't how Tim thought he would be spending the evening; he couldn't rectify it in his head.

"Why are they being nice to me? What do they want from me?" he thought to himself.

A rarity in Wakefield, the restaurant sat almost empty, just the three of them, apart from a couple of servers and one chef who watched them eagerly through the pass.

The eatery's aesthetic was a blend of street food with a fine dining twist. In his youth, Tim had passed through more service industry jobs than he had wanted to, but there was something about overpaid, lazy management and people's comfort with disrespecting servers that always irked him.

He had been let go more than once for bouncing a rude customer off the floor. How he had made it into the army with his disdain for taking orders, he would never really know.

Norman sat with a newspaper on his lap. "Local journalist acquitted of murder count," it printed in huge letters. The story had gripped and divided the town due to its controversial nature, causing a widespread debate that would linger long after the parties involved would be happy with.

"Bar fight erupts, one dead." Another headline; for a town so known for its beauty and peace, Wakefield had been marred with scandal as of late.

"How long are you in town for?" Norman asked, watching Tim intently. He could see the discomfort in Tim as he sat there. He noticed Tim's eyes scanning the room, checking for exits and watching over his shoulder for passersby.

"When I came home, I couldn't adjust. It didn't feel normal. It wasn't long ago I was on patrol, gun in hand. I was scared, of course, but I felt the comfort of having my brothers around me. Then before you know it, I'm an old man! Sometimes, all it would take is a car backfiring or a firework, and there I am again, back there. You aren't alone, son. You may have left the battlefield, but I don't think you ever left the war. Right here, now, you aren't alone, son. Do you understand what I'm trying to tell you?"

Tim didn't know these people; he didn't trust them. He knew there wasn't a reason for it, but looking into Norman's eyes, he could see history and experience, but also empathy. This was a man whom the world had not been kind to—cruel, even—but yet he still smiled, thanked the waiters with a cheeky grin, tipped every single time without fail, and no matter how bad things seemed, he never lost that spark in his eyes.

The rest of the night was spent like that; they traded stories over coffee and just laughed. Luke listened eagerly to every story, even the ones he had heard a thousand times. He knew the importance of words and the power they had; he took nothing said for granted.

When you are forced to grow up at such a young age, you treat the world differently, sometimes to your detriment. Luke rarely spent time with those his age and reveled in a good story.

Something became apparent very early: Luke never spoke of his mum. He had no bad words for her—no negative thoughts that he would express out loud, anyway. His dad was his world, his hero.

"Big man!" a voice shouted, bursting through the door and making his way straight to the front of the counter. Young and brash, this man stood tall and confident. He paid no attention to his surroundings and cared little for what others thought of him; that was clear very early on. Tim's eyes fixed on him instantly.

"Watch it, old boy," the young man said to Norman, almost knocking him out of his chair on his way through.

And just like that, the shaking in Tim's hands, the anxiety, and the panic had gone.

Sometimes you leave the battleground; sometimes it comes to you.

Tim watched the young lad, observing his intent and demeanor. He wanted to see if this young man meant any harm or if he was just loud. Being old enough to understand intent better than most, Tim liked to think this young man meant no harm.

"You got a staring problem, old man?" the young man yelled across the café.

Some things don't always work out how you expect them to, though. His eyes fixed on Tim, and Tim's eyes locked onto him. Norman ushered Luke toward the door, staying calm. You can tell a lot about a man by how he acts under stress or pressure. Norman didn't flinch, not for a second.

"Hey, Tim, time to go, yeah? We don't need this; Luke doesn't need to see this."

And like that, Tim was back on Earth. He knew Norm was right; there was no need to escalate the situation further than it had gone, a perspective gained more with age.

In his youth, Tim would have rushed in headfirst— to hell with the consequences! He wouldn't have given a second thought to those he hurt, including himself. More than once, he had to stitch himself up or ice swollen knuckles. He knew Norman was right: blood is never worth the price of pride.

Tim looked back over the shoulder of the young man at the waiters and waitresses, gauging their reactions. The last thing he would allow himself to do was leave if he felt like he was leaving someone in a position they didn't want to be in. To him, not doing anything to help was just as bad as the act committed.

As they walked along the beach, making their way home, Tim struggled to let go of the situation back at the café.

"It takes a good man to swallow his pride and know when to walk away," Norm said quietly, watching Tim's face as he still tried to make sense of the evening.

He knew Norm was right, but that didn't make the situation easier. Tim recognized he was overthinking and perhaps overreacting, but letting sleeping dogs lie had never been for him.

He stopped to watch the waves crash against the rocks across the water, taking a second to close his eyes, feel the cold air brush over him, and just breathe.

Tim's moment of tranquility was cut short by the sound of quick shuffling steps on the wooden decking beneath him. He opened his eyes to see the young lad from the café making a beeline toward him. Crouched slightly, the boy kept one hand behind his back, trying to hide something he had been holding.

Taking no chances, Tim moved aside, stepped back, and threw a knee straight down the middle, knocking the young man back. As he fell, the knife he had tried to conceal bounced out of his hand and across the floor. Tim quickly picked up the knife and tossed it as far away as he could before taking a step toward his attacker and throwing another knee.

The young lad, seeing his weapon gone and realizing very quickly that this was not a fight he was winning, scrambled to his feet and ran off into the night.

"Hey!" Luke called out. "You good?"

Taking a breath, Tim shot him a quick thumbs-up, keeping an eye on the path the young lad had taken.

Walking back into his hotel that night felt strange for Tim. He looked at the pills laid out on the floor and the empty bottles of whiskey left lying about. The room was empty, and he was alone...but in a way, he had always been, until tonight.

Tim reached down, picked up the last half-empty bottle of whiskey, and brought it to his lips. He could smell the spices, the oak, and the alcohol. He raised the bottle slowly, contemplating throwing it in the bin, ashamed to waste good whiskey.

Hours later, he awoke in the night, rolling over to check on Hannah before the horror of realization dawned on him: she wasn't there. There was no warmth or comfort. He would roll over in the night, watch her sleeping peacefully, kiss his thumb, and place it on her cheek so as not to wake her. He took comfort in her presence.

But now, he was alone. "I hope there's whiskey left," he thought to himself, running his hand along the empty bed space.

His mind was taken back to a time when things were simpler. Before she left, it felt like she was the only person on the planet. The stresses and pressures from the day didn't seem to matter; he would clock in to work and know that in eight hours, he'd be home and back in her arms, and nothing else would matter.

Of course, they would fight and argue like couples do, but it never bothered him. "If I'm going to wake up next to anyone, it would only ever be you. If I'm going to feel anyone's heart, it's going to be yours. And if I'm going to argue with anyone, there's no one on this planet I would rather argue with than you," he would tell her.

It's something lost in today's society, but he never took her criticism or their arguments to heart. He never let words said in anger affect him or linger because he knew that if she was willing to stay and argue with him, it meant she cared. It was the day the arguing stopped that he knew it was over.

Tim pulled himself up and made his way out into the cold night air. It was funny how the quietest rooms could be the loudest sometimes.

CHAPTER 9

"**P**eople sleep peaceably in their beds at night only because rough men stand ready to do violence on their behalf."
– George Orwell –

"Last tour, Sergeant?" a voice called out loudly over the helicopter blades that seemed to fill the air. Tim just nodded; he knew his time in the army was coming to an end. Hannah waited patiently at home, and the thought was enough. The time for violence and bloodshed was over. He wasn't needed anymore. He had made it through this tour without firing a single round of ammunition and had hoped to keep it that way.

In life, we don't always get what we want. Tim made his way through the town, gun in hand, accompanied by Malik, a third-generation soldier who had been shadowing him for a while. Malik was young and strong, with jet-black hair that had streaks of gray running down into his beard. Malik's father had served with Tim before retiring and had trusted Tim with his life on more than one occasion. Wanting to make his dad proud, Malik reveled in serving alongside him.

They made their way through the town, passing the markets and fishing spots, stopping to admire the beautiful orange sunrise that encapsulated the town, the clouds like artwork. Malik took a moment to thank God with a smile, and they carried on.

Then, all of a sudden, screams began filling the air. Tim unholstered his weapon and, without a second thought, began running towards the screams.

"My son!" a young woman begged Tim, holding in her arms a young boy whose throat had been cut from ear to ear. Her clothes were soaked in red, washed away only by her tears. Malik had thrown himself down, and before anyone could grasp the situation, he had already called in a medic. He knelt, holding a rag he had stolen from a nearby table to stem the bleeding, one hand pressed against the young lad's neck, listening for a pulse.

"Who did this?" Tim asked. The crying woman pointed in the direction, and he took off, running at full speed, desperate to find the man who could commit such a heinous act. The assailant had covered his face but, in his attack, had nicked an artery of the young lad, leaving a trail of blood that Tim followed with vicious intent.

He lunged at the man before being thrown down to the ground, feeling a burning sensation course through his abdomen. He knew instantly he had been stabbed. His body became cold and clammy as his lungs tightened, and he fell to the ground.

He watched the man realize what he had done. He knew he had to kill Tim; he couldn't let him survive. Picking up the blade he had dropped in the scramble, he made his way back toward Tim, smiling as he did. Tim felt the cold steel against his neck and closed his eyes.

"I'm sorry, Han," he whispered to himself, picturing her smile for the last time. If this was to be his final moment, he would pass how he always intended—with her in his mind.

Suddenly, he felt the cold steel move away. He opened his eyes to see Malik, who had come running through like a bat out of hell, charging at the attacker and smashing his head onto the concrete as he fell.

Tim desperately tried to pull himself to his feet, feeling the blood pulse with every beat of his heart; he didn't have long.

"Stop, please! I surrender!" the attacker pleaded, dropping to his knees and raising his hands into the air. Malik reached for his gun to aim at the assailant, hoping to buy enough time to cuff him, but he realized, in the scuffle, that he had dropped it.

He turned his head to find it before the attacker pulled a knife from his boot and drove it straight into Malik's neck. Malik fell onto his back, clutching his neck. He looked over to Tim, his eyes welling with tears; he had let Tim down. He had let his dad down.

The man stood up, looked Malik in the eyes, put one hand on the back of his head, and plunged the knife slowly through his heart. Malik fought desperately, pressing his hands against the attacker, pleading quietly, but it meant nothing.

The assailant reveled in seeing Malik suffer, watching deep into his eyes as blood slowly poured from Malik's mouth. He held his head up before angling it toward Tim. He wanted Tim to watch; he wanted him to see the light go out in Malik's eyes. As the knife pierced his heart, Malik let out a single gargle of blood, and just like that, he was gone.

Malik fell, his eyes still fixed on Tim.

"I surrender," he said, throwing the knife to the ground and dropping to his knees, a smile now beaming ear to ear. Tim pulled himself to his feet and moved toward the attacker, who had both hands in front of him.

"Arrest me," the man smirked, looking deep into Tim's eyes.

Tim unholstered his gun, removed the clip, and began smashing the attacker in the head repeatedly, not stopping even when he felt brain matter and bone soaking his hands. He felt his breath slipping away with every strike, but that didn't matter. This bastard would know he had messed up, and Tim wasn't going to relent for a second. By the time he finished, it was hard to tell what was left of the attacker. They would later find out that the young lad had survived, leaving nothing but a scar across his neck.

The reason behind two lives being lost that day, though, remained a mystery—something that would haunt Tim for the rest of his life.

Tim took a second, struggling to regain his breath. He looked down at his hands, dripping with blood. He flicked the butt of the gun to throw off the excess flaps of skin and brain matter onto the floor; it was impossible at this point to tell whose blood was whose. He looked over at Malik's lifeless body, the blood from his wound still pumping. Anxiety and guilt filled his chest, and his head spun. His last memory was of Malik's head hitting the ground, looking into his eyes.

The last thing crossing his mind before everything went black was Hannah; he prayed that she knew how much he loved her.

Tim lay unconscious for three days as doctors and nurses worked tirelessly around him. Hannah never once left his side. She watched medical professionals come and go, witnessed them open him up and stitch him back together more times than she could count, and she cleaned him and took care of him without a single complaint.

He had been airlifted home after becoming stable and had remained comatose since. Hannah sat by Tim, stroking his black and grey hair. She ran her hand along his chest, feeling his heart beating slowly. She held his hands and listened to his breathing. Tim's hands were rough and bruised. She wasn't sure what had happened fully, but the bruising on his hands, forearms, and face, along with the large stitches running across his abdomen—at least thirty—made it clear he had been through hell. Not for the first time, but he had never been out this long.

He always came back! She begged and pleaded with God.

"He has to come back." Tears streamed down her cheeks.

"I love you this big," she would sing, their song. She sang it to him, usually throwing her arms out and trying to get him to dance. Tim never missed an opportunity to take Hannah by the hand and hold her.

"I'm not leaving you! I'm here, I'm right here!" She squeezed his hand tightly, trying with everything she had to stop the welling in her eyes, which had already been burnt from crying.

The conversations with doctors discussing what to do if he didn't wake up filled her with dread. She wasn't prepared for this; she had a life planned out with Tim! She had never dared to tell him for fear of losing him, but she knew when he was there. Something she had always valued in Tim was that he was present. In every moment together, he was there; he paid attention to the little things and listened not only to her words but also to her actions.

She thought back to the first time she got ill around Tim. She had told him to run for the hills, to save himself. But he didn't falter for a second. Before she knew it, she was neck-deep in hot water bottles and blankets. He took every step possible to make sure she was looked after and felt loved and safe at every turn.

It wasn't just the things he could provide; to her, his presence felt like home. It was as if the world could fall apart at any moment, and she knew they would be okay.

What hurt more was knowing that Tim had saved her at every possible moment. He had cared for her at times when she didn't even want it, when she felt like she didn't deserve it. She had never understood why she was so important to Tim. She loved him, of course, but she struggled to understand how she deserved a love like this.

Tim would always shoot her a slight smile and a wink, telling her, "With a bum like that, how could I not?"

She hurt knowing all of this and realizing that in this moment, there was nothing she could do. There was no saving the day, no last-minute fix like those superhero movies he had loved.

It was the only time; time would be the deciding factor here. As time tends to do, it would make or break this life for both of them.

"I brought coffee," a voice whispered from the doorway. Sam, the best friend, shot Tim a look to see if he was awake before stepping in and handing Hannah the drink. He looked into her eyes, reached over, and placed a hand on her shoulder, brushing her hair out of her face and over one of her ears. He didn't say much; he just watched Tim, studying him. They had never liked each other. Tim didn't trust him, not for a second. He had known men like this—like worms that burrow under your skin. Despite this, Hannah trusted him, so that was it; he wouldn't say another word.

"Come on, you need fresh air. It'll do you the world of good," he pleaded.

Tim's eyes flickered; the lights from the room blinded him. He listened to the world around him; he could hear the monitors beeping, the noise from the ventilation almost deafening.

Opening his eyes, he saw Sam leading Hannah out of the room, his hand around her waist guiding her.

He awoke alone.

Tim's memory was fuzzy. He pulled at the tubes around him, starting with the one in his nose. It felt like it had clawed its way into his brain. Next, he grabbed whatever had been in his arms; he hated needles. Blood poured down his arm as he pulled himself out of the bed.

"Hey, hey, hey!" a voice called, rushing in.

He ignored the poor nurse as he tried to pull himself to his feet, but nothing worked. His legs didn't respond. Had he been out that long? The large nurse wrapped her arms around him and pulled him back onto the bed, scrambling to fix the open wounds on his arm, not realizing that when he stood, he had pulled the stitching from his stomach.

"Where's Hannah?" he asked through pained breaths.

"Your friend has just left; her boyfriend took her to get some fresh air."

That cut like a knife, he thought to himself. Poor timing on his part.

Tim laid back down. Everything hurt; his entire body felt like it had been opened by a razor. The last few days had been a blur of pain, and his memory was now just chunks of what happened, nothing solid.

"Malik?" he asked the nurse.

Realizing what Tim had just asked, she looked at him with sorrow in her eyes. She knew, but how could she tell him?

"Everything is going to be okay," she said, pulling a pillow up behind his head before leaving.

Tim watched the sunset through the window, observing the orange and red hues that engulfed the sky like flames. He watched it dissipate into a sky full of stars.

He thought about the passage of time, a career filled with bloodshed and shell casings, and wondered if any of it meant anything. Had he ever really left a place better than it was before he arrived?

But he knew now, at this moment, that the fight was over for him. He was no good anymore, and there was nothing left for him to give. He looked at his hands, at the scarring along his knuckles.

"Whose hands are these?" he thought to himself. They were his hands, but older, more wrinkled than they had ever been, with calluses built up around the bottoms of his fingers. He could see a small reflection of his face in the window: wrinkles around his eyes and the grey in his hair becoming clearer by the day. He looked just like his father. He was older than his dad had ever been.

He thought back to the last time he had seen his father: the open casket, the pale face, and the cold skin. He rested his hand on his heart, but there was no beat. He forgave him at that moment; he knew their battle was over.

Tim always thought they had one bout left in them maybe that would solve it. But he knew in life they would never come to terms; there was too much history, too much violence, and maybe they were too much alike. His mum never looked at him the same after his father's passing. She never had to say it, but he knew that every time she looked at him, all she saw was the man she loved—a memory of a man no longer here on this mortal plane. He never blamed her for this, despite how much it hurt. Tim just prayed his father found the peace in death that he never found in life.

As the temperature dropped that night, Tim laid there listening to the world moving outside. He listened to the sounds of ambulances and the hustle of the busy city streets die down into hushed tones, and he listened to the music flowing through the streets from the local clubs. There was something about city life that Tim loved; it grounded him, kept him humble.

In his youth, he would look at the towering buildings in awe, amazed at the different lives people seemed to live here, how much faster-paced everyone was. Nobody stopped to savor the moment, enjoy the night sky, or listen to the birds tweeting.

"When you live as lonely as I have, it's easier to appreciate the little things," he thought to himself.

As the night wore on, Tim's memories came slowly trickling back. He knew Malik hadn't made it; he knew he would have to speak to his father and explain how it happened, how he failed.

Had he been younger, would he have been able to stop this from happening? Had he missed a step? He knew better than to live on "ifs" and "buts," but that didn't stop the guilt from tearing his insides out, from breaking his heart.

He closed his eyes, took a breath, and let sleep consume him.

Tim awoke to the sound of giggling; he would know that laugh in any room. He could hear Hannah.

"Would your boyfriend like a coffee?" the nurse asked.

"No, thank you," she replied, getting up and making her way across the hospital room to take Tim by the hand. One hand rested on his forearm; she always held it when she felt nervous or uncomfortable.

"Are you going to tell that lovely nurse that smiley dickhead is not your partner at any point?" he thought to himself. He wasn't going to bring that up; he had thought about picking his battles, but he lost the last one, and he knew he wouldn't win this one.

Hannah pulled a chair as close to the bed as she could and rested her head on Tim's chest, avoiding the cut running along his abdomen, just listening to his heartbeat. It was like music. When she got the call that he had been stabbed, she could barely stand; her legs felt like jelly, and her hands shook, almost dropping the phone. She battled her own body, trying to stay upright; she wanted to crumble and break, but she knew he wouldn't.

She knew she wasn't in any state to drive, so she had asked Sam to take her. Not her first choice, nor her second or third, but in desperation, she had reached out. Panicked, she spent the entire journey thinking; she knew he was stable, but not seeing it with her own eyes made her mind her own worst enemy.

She held in all the fear and panic while rushing up the hospital stairs. She raced to be by his side, only breaking when she saw him lying still, doctors and nurses rushing around him, trying to put him back together. She saw one nurse covered in blood from head to toe.

"Is that all his?" she thought.

Seeing the tubes and the machines firing, everything inside her broke. He was the strongest person she knew—her protector, her guardian. How could he be hurt?

"I'll never let anyone hurt me because I've got something to come home to that they don't," he would tell her.

"What's that?" she would ask, her big brown eyes melting his heart.

"You! There's not a man on this planet that could stop me from getting home to you. You are every beat of my heart, and I promise you, I'll always come home."

But this wasn't coming home, not how he had promised.

She watched his body convulse.

"We're losing him..." a nurse shouted firmly, ushering another to remove her from the room.

"No!" she screamed as the machine flat lined before she was pulled out.

Sitting there, listening to his heartbeat, was everything in this moment; nothing else mattered.

"I love you this big," Tim whispered, running his hand through her hair.

Feeling Tim's hand and hearing his voice, Hannah let out a gasp and melted her head into his soft chest. Breaking down, she just sobbed, squeezing him as hard as she ever had in her entire life. She grabbed one of his arms and pulled it tight over herself with all her might, relief washing through her as she was finally able to let go of every stress from the last few days.

Between sleep deprivation and stress, she knew she was a mess; she had cried so much that her eyes ran a bright shade of red, and she hadn't eaten. How could she?

"You're beautiful," he told her, lifting his head to look into her eyes.

He was home.

CHAPTER 10

"I may not have gone where I intended to go, but I think I have ended up where I needed to be."
- Douglas Adams -

Tim made his way across the cold beach, clutching a whiskey bottle in his hands like a weapon he was ready to fire. He stood where the water met the sand, feeling the cold water wash over his feet, and took a deep sip of whiskey, the burn searing his throat. He swayed with the wind and listened to the music of the sea, the cold breeze running through his hair.

"Mr. T?" a small voice called out.

He looked around and saw Luke standing there, shivering in the cold.

"Are you okay?" Luke asked nervously.

Tim took a step back, noticing the fear in Luke's eyes. He scanned Tim anxiously, sensing that something was wrong but unsure how to ask or what to do. A poor young child forced to grow up quickly in a world he did not understand—Tim knew this feeling all too well. So why did he feel like he was only adding to it?

"Is everything okay?" Tim asked quietly, moving the bottle behind his back.

"I saw you from my window. I was worried about you."

"Where's your dad?"

"He fell asleep on the deck."

"Let's get you home," Tim said, turning around and launching the almost empty bottle into the sea before leading Luke home.

As they walked up the deck, Tim saw Norman sleeping, his flat cap covering his eyes. He reached under him, picked him up, and carried him through the house and upstairs, placing him gently into bed. Luke didn't leave his side for a second.

There was only so much Tim could do for his dad. He knew how to give him medication, when to roll him over, and how to change him, but he wasn't strong enough to pick Norman up when he fell. The number of times he had laid on the floor with his hands under his dad's head to stop it from bouncing off the floor was countless.

Tim made his way downstairs and looked at the mess on the floor: empty food boxes and cobwebs building up in the corners. This was no way to live.

"Hey, you hungry?"

Luke just nodded.

"What have you got in?" Tim asked.

It dawned on Tim very quickly that there wasn't any food. The empty boxes, the cupboards, and the fridge held nothing—not a tin or a box in sight. He learned that night when his mum left, she took everything—everything she could. Luke had been forced to grow up overnight; he didn't know how to cook or clean properly. This was all new to him. He would wake early to give his dad his medication and look after him, but he only knew how to do that from watching carers come and go. No one had ever stopped to ask him, to check on him.

Norman woke that morning to the smell of cooked food floating down the halls—the smell of grilled turkey and eggs. For a second, he wondered if he was having a stroke.

Tim had spent the night cleaning and fixing broken doors, beginning a serious battle with the spider army that had grown very fond of their new home. Stick in hand, Norman made his way down the now dirt-free stairs. Whose home had he woken in?

It broke his heart every day that he couldn't do the little things he liked, like he used to. One time that broke his heart was seeing the front garden slowly taken over by weeds. Growing up, his mother, a florist, had taken great pride in teaching her son not just the things he needed to be a man, but how to turn a house into a home—something he had taken great pride in once upon a time.

He looked at Tim; something was different—he was... sober?

It's amazing what a little kindness will do to a person.

He saw Luke asleep on the sofa and couldn't remember the last time he had seen his son at such peace.

"How long has he been asleep for?" Norman asked, running his hands through his son's long ginger hair.

"Hours," Tim smiled.

"And the cleaning?"

"I wanted to thank you."

"For what?"

"Treating me... like a human," he said, pulling a hot tray out of the oven and placing it down. The smell of fresh food filled the air.

Norman sat down as Tim slipped a fresh cup of coffee in front of him.

"When did you have time to get all of this?" Norman asked, lifting the cup to smell the coffee.

"It's Wakefield; there's always something open."

Waking up for Luke that morning brought a feeling he couldn't describe. For the first time in a long time, there was color in the house, the light looked brighter, and the fresh Hoover carpet! He couldn't describe it, but he woke for the first time in a long time without worrying.

"I can't afford to hire you," Norman joked, although he would have if he could, he thought to himself.

Norm watched Tim as he shifted his eyes about the kitchen, looking for things to clean, for something to keep his mind occupied.

"You can relax, sir," he whispered, observing Tim's hands shake. He could see the effect that not drinking for one night had on him, and he knew the next few days were going to be more brutal than Tim could ever imagine.

Alcohol withdrawal symptoms take around eight hours to start. Eight hours—that's crazy, right? That's one night's sleep separating you from drinking and the onset of cold sweats, nausea, vomiting, and anxiety.

CHAPTER 11

"Thou shalt not be a victim, thou shalt not be a perpe-trator, but, above all, thou shalt not be a bystander."
- Yehuda Bauer -

Running his hands through Hannah's hair, Tim felt a sense of peace he hadn't experienced in a long time. Much to the dismay of the nurses, he had wiggled himself as far over the bed as he could, and Hannah had scooched in beside him.

Twenty-four hours ago, she thought she had lost him, and she wasn't going to waste a second here.

He held her chin up toward him and looked into her eyes, running his fingers along her beautiful red lips. He savored the details of her face, and she would catch him staring at her.

"What?" she would giggle.

"I like your face," he would say, smiling back. Every time he did, she would pout, and he would pull her in a little tighter, squeezing until he heard her let out a little laugh that would melt his heart. That same laugh echoed in his mind; he lived for it. Tim would bury his hand in his chest and rip his heart straight out if it meant getting to hear that laugh one last time.

"Babe, I brought you food," Sam said loudly, bursting into the hospital room.

"Babe?" Tim whispered. Hannah chuckled, slapping him on the chest in jest and hopping out of bed.

"Sorry, Timothy, I didn't think you'd be up for eating, so I didn't buy you anything," Sam said, smirking at Tim when Hannah looked away, tilting his head to check out her backside as she walked back toward the bed.

As Hannah looked down into the bag, rummaging for food, Tim dropped his smile and looked deep into Sam's eyes. Anger burned red as he stared into Sam's soul. Sam had felt comfortable messing with Tim while he was bed-bound, but something about the look Tim shot him turned his legs to jelly. His hands began trembling as his bladder slowly released something he probably wished it hadn't.

Tim just smiled as Hannah handed him a half-ripped burger she had split with her hands, watching with a grin as Sam shot out of the room.

"What's up with him?"

"Think he needed a piss," Tim chuckled.

Hannah just shrugged and carried on eating.

Tim knew Sam; he knew men like that—opportunists, smiley and corrupt. But he was stupid, wearing every emotion on his face. He would never punish Hannah by making her feel dumb for not noticing it. She had a good heart, and that was something Tim adored. He loved how much she cared about people.

How she would run back into the shops if it meant grabbing food for the homeless who congregated outside, or how she would stop to pet every dog—he loved how much she cared. He had told her a thousand times that she was one of the very few people on the entire planet who was just as beautiful on the outside as she was on the inside, and he would kill and die a thousand times to protect that.

Sam walked back in, and his face had changed. The look of fear was gone, replaced by a wry smile that made Tim uneasy. Tim understood the danger of stupidity.

"Hey, I've got to go. Do you need a lift?" Sam asked, grabbing his things.

Hannah popped up. Little did Tim know, she had been moving the flat around for his return. She had rearranged the TV in a way that resembled a small cinema. She could barely contain her excitement, knowing Tim was home for good, but she had to finish everything before he was discharged. Popping up, she kissed Tim—electric—pulling him toward her tightly.

"One more day," she said, smiling.

"Hey, did you change your trousers?" she asked Sam as they left the room. Before the door shut, Sam turned and gave a smile to Tim that turned his stomach. He didn't know what Sam planned, but he recognized evil, and Sam wore it clear as day.

That look didn't sit right with him. He tried to get comfortable, not to think about it, and to avoid letting these negative thoughts eat away at him, but it was in his head and wasn't going anywhere now.

Tim got himself up and pulled the tubing from his arms, ignoring the small squirts of blood that escaped when he did. He grabbed whatever clothing Hannah had left for him and made his way for the door, ignoring the nurses who called for him. The anxiety built up inside him, and he couldn't let it go; he had to leave.

Tim flagged down the first taxi he could find.

"Can I borrow your phone, sir?" he asked, hovering over the back seat.

He called and called, but nobody answered until...

"Sorry, Hannah's a little busy," Sam chuckled over the phone before the line cut out.

"FUCK!" Tim exclaimed.

He pulled his shirt up to look at the stitching. At some point, leaving the hospital, he had pulled something loose and could feel the blood trickling down. It felt right, like something had been twisting his insides.

This wasn't helping his nerves; he felt like his insides had been ripped in half as his heart raced. He watched helplessly outside the window of the taxi.

"Come on, come on," he thought. Rain poured down the windows as he paced as much as he could.

The car came to a halt, and Tim jumped out, throwing the driver whatever cash he had on him without thinking. He hit the ground running straight for the lobby, bursting through the front door and making his way up the stairs. With every step, he felt his knife wound opening a little more, but he ignored the burning that became more intense.

He nearly fell near the top; the burning was almost too much to bear as he fell forward and clutched his side, struggling to breathe. He felt his consciousness fading as he fought to move, feeling as though he had been stabbed all over again.

Tim put a hand down to catch himself at the top of the landing and took a deep breath as he closed his eyes. His whole body tensed up, and he felt his blood pressure drop, his skin turning pale and clammy.

"Not again," he thought to himself.

His head spun, and the world began to fade when, all of a sudden, he heard a blood-curdling scream echo through the entire building—a shriek that hit him like a shot of adrenaline. That was Hannah's voice.

He punched the side of his abdomen; the pain was so severe that it snapped him awake, and he took off, bursting through the front door and almost taking it off its hinges.

Blood splattered on the floor and walls! Posters had been knocked down, and Hannah's ripped top lay on the floor.

"Hannah!" he screamed, making his way through their flat.

Hannah let out another scream. Tim burst through the door to their bedroom, and there it was: blood sprayed across her face, her nose was broken, the nasal bone poking through the flesh. He had hit her, and he had hit her hard! Her right eye had swollen shut, and her lips were split, but it hadn't stopped her from fighting. Under her fingernails were chunks of flesh from where, in an attempt to fight him off, she had gouged at whatever bits of skin she could find. She used every limb desperately trying to push him off of her, her knees pressed against his chest as he attempted to pull his trousers down.

Tim grabbed Sam and threw him across the room, tripping him over his trousers.

"Whoa, it is not what it looks like," he pleaded.

"She wanted this! She wanted what you couldn't give her. She told me, and she's loved it every single fucking time you've been away." Sam squirmed, trying to pull up his trousers. He saw the blood pouring down Tim's stomach, and as he reached down to grab his trousers, he lunged forward and dug his fingers straight into Tim's wound, pushing as hard as he could with his thumb and twisting it.

Sam pulled his thumb out as hard as he could, pulling whatever pieces of flesh he could and tearing out the remaining stitches before jamming his fingers back in. Screaming in agony, Tim threw him to the ground, one hand gripping his throat as tight as possible before lifting his leg and smashing it down into Sam's face!

Sam raised both his hands as if to surrender, but it was too late!

Tim smashed and smashed, ignoring the cracking of Sam's skull!

Hannah watched in absolute horror! She wanted to scream and ask Tim to stop, but the words wouldn't come out of her mouth. She pawed at the clothes around her, trying to cover herself up.

"Fuck you, cunt!" he screamed, still smashing! Sam's arms slapped against Tim's feet, trying with pure desperation to stop him before they fell.

Sam's arms fell by his side as he gurgled blood, spitting it out in a desperate attempt to breathe; his one eye darting around before glazing over. Between convulsions and spurts of blood, he would pass away that evening. He lasted longer than the paramedics thought he would, but they theorized that even if he had survived, he would have lived the rest of his life brain dead anyway, as chunks of his brain lay scattered across the floor while Tim turned to check on Hannah.

She was crying! Her vision blurred as she reached out, and when Tim grabbed her, she pushed him away.

"Hey, baby, it's me," he said. Before he finished the sentence, she had grabbed him as hard as possible while he wrapped his arms around her.

"It's over, I'm here!" he repeated.

"You're safe! You are loved!"

Hannah buried her face in Tim's chest and sobbed.

"It's all my fault," she tried to say through her whimpers.

"Nothing is your fault at all! Hey, don't you dare..." He squeezed her hard as she ran her hands along his arms, and then Hannah felt his skin go cold.

"Baby?" she asked.

"Baby?"

Tim fell back off the bed, smashing his head on the wooden bed frame and falling unconscious. His skin had gone cold and clammy, and his wounds had become too much to bear. She was safe; that's all that mattered. In that moment, he was ready to die knowing she was okay; nothing else mattered more to him.

Hannah jumped over the bed and grabbed Tim, wrapping her arms around him tightly.

"Please wake up," she begged, patting his face and shaking him as hard as she could. She didn't know what to do.

Her phone had been lost all evening, so she reached into Tim's pockets. With one hand, she called an ambulance, and with the other, she clutched Tim.

"Please stay with me! Please don't leave me," she whispered, her heart breaking.

CHAPTER 12

"Amid winter, I found there was, within me, an invincible summer. And that makes me happy. For it says that no matter how hard the world pushes against me, within me, there's something stronger — something better, pushing right back."

• Albert Camus -

Dear Dad,

There are a few things I want to clear up. Firstly, I need to apologise; I wasn't always the best son, and more than that, I was a horrible son! Now, don't get me wrong, I'm not going to lie and say you were any better as a father, but that's no excuse for how I treated you.

I often wonder if I hadn't pushed you away, would we have ever found a way to get along? Hell, maybe if you had better people around you, you would still be here.

We can't change the past; I know you would if you could. And I know how much it broke you when Mum left. None of us would ever really know how much.

You taught me everything I know. You taught me how to be a man, and how to stand up when it matters. You showed me the importance of empathy. I still crack jokes when the world feels like it is falling apart; you taught me the importance of making people happy, especially when they didn't feel like they would ever smile again.

I'm sorry those demons got the best of you. But I have to let go of the past now; I have to let go of everything that happened because if I stop for too long and think about it—everything you did, everything I did—I think I would break.

So, I'm saying goodbye for now. I can't lie and say that when we meet again, punches won't be thrown, but laughs will be, too. No one could make me laugh like you did.

I hope you know... you were my hero.

Until we meet again.

T.

CHAPTER 13

Tim sat alone, pen in hand, scribbling to himself. He had begun these writings as a final goodbye, but the more he wrote and the longer he spent here, the more it became a sort of therapy.

That morning, he had sat with Norman and Luke, having breakfast. They had gone back and forth, jesting between themselves, enjoying coffee, and just laughing. It had been so long since he had laughed like that; it felt strange. But for the first time in a long time, he had found a strange kind of peace.

"You good?" Norm asked, slowly walking out with his walking stick in hand. Tim gave him a nod and stood to pull a chair out for Norman to sit down in.

They looked across the beach, the blue sky lighting up the morning ocean, the waves still under the bright sky. Before long, a figure walked past—hood up, hat down—and for a moment, it stopped to stare at Tim.

"Is that..." Norm asked. Tim said nothing; he took a sip of his coffee and smiled at Norm.

"It's not worth it," he said, relaxing in his chair.

"I was thinking about what you said about your front garden. I know you hate seeing it like that, but I was just wondering if you wanted me to take a crack at it," Tim asked, still leaning back in his chair and watching the hooded figure walk off in the distance.

"You've already done more than we could have ever asked for," Norm said, tears welling up in his eyes. Norm had struggled to adjust to this life—confined and restricted. He still felt eighteen most days until he looked in the mirror or tried moving.

Every night before he went to bed, he would look across his bedroom at the photo of himself and his wife taken on their wedding day, thinking back to their youth. When he proposed, he was twenty-six and had taken her to a place simply called Paradise, a clifftop surrounded by trees but visible through one small walkway. This walkway was positioned just right so that if you got there at the right time of day, the sun would shine off the water and straight up to where you would be seated.

He took her there, blindfolded her, and when she took it off, he had her read this giant card he had folded up and hidden. She read it out loud, and he had written a beautiful piece describing what she meant to him. He told her how every single day her mere presence brought him joy that he didn't think existed in today's world. At the bottom of the note, he wrote, "Look down." When she did, there he knelt... ring in hand.

He would never forget her face as she pulled her hands up over her mouth—something she had joked about previously, never understanding why women did that. Now she did.

They embraced and, in that moment, knew they would be together forever. It's a nice thought, anyway. Norm never got over his love—his wife, the mother of his child—leaving. He had trouble explaining this to Luke, but Luke never really asked; his main concern was seeing his dad's health deteriorate. Norm never blamed her; he felt his health declining as he got older and would never have asked anyone to bear that responsibility.

Would he have done it for her? In a million lifetimes, he would every single time. But he understood that what he struggled with was her leaving in the dead of night, never saying a word, no explanation. When someone passes, we mourn their loss—the loss they couldn't control. We don't blame them, but when someone leaves, it's a different feeling.

Norm wanted to drink himself to death; he wanted to break, give up, scream up to God, and ask why someone so perfect could come into his life only to disappear. But he sat across from Luke and knew that what he wanted didn't matter. He had to be strong; he had to be present, and he wasn't going to fail his son.

Tim had always found he was best when he kept busy. He never felt comfortable sitting around; something about it made him feel lazy. When Hannah left, he occupied his time by working every hour he could, and he found things around the flat that needed fixing. Gardening had always been a strange one for him—oddly therapeutic. He was happy enough, content even, knowing there were goals and jobs ahead that he could focus on in his mind, and that's what he did. He reveled in it.

As much as Norman could do, he would, but he knew he wasn't as spry as he once was. Norm had boxed in his youth;

he always had this dream of teaching Luke as he got older, and knowing that this was not something he would ever fulfill himself broke him inside.

As the drink cleared Tim's system, it didn't take long for the shakes to start and the fever to set in. He had left a number with Luke and made his way back to the hotel, knowing he had to sweat the alcohol out of his system. It wouldn't be easy; he knew that.

Walking into the hotel room that night, everything was silent. He felt a calmness that he hadn't experienced in a long time. But it wouldn't take long for the shakes to hit his body like an earthquake. He fell to his knees, clutching his scar in pain. Why had that started burning? He felt like he had been stabbed all over again.

Tim ran across the room, pulled the bin bag out of the bin, and threw up straight into the empty plastic container. He fell, his back sliding down the wall, and for a moment, he just sat there, focusing on his breath.

"Hello, son," a voice called out—a voice he hadn't heard in a very long time.

"Dad?"

"I'm hallucinating! You're dead!" he screamed.

But there he stood, all five foot eleven, with brown hair and blue eyes looking at Tim. He could see the freckles on his cheeks, clear as the day he died. Tim pulled himself to his feet. Looking into his dad's brown eyes, he felt like a child again.

"I'm sorry," Tim said quietly, his eyes welling.

His dad said nothing; he just looked at him with a wistful smile before disappearing. Tim's head spun as he clutched at anything around him, trying to keep his balance, but nothing worked. It was too late; he could feel himself falling. He hit the ground with a crash, knocking himself unconscious.

Tim lay on the floor, blood trickling from his nose, his face pressed into the carpet. He closed his eyes, hoping to stop the spinning when he saw a pair of feet move past him. He turned his head to look up, and there stood Mike...his brother.

"What the fuck is happening?" Mike stood there, pale-faced, with bright green eyes, wearing the same blue button-up he had been in the day he took his life.

Tim dropped to his knees and pleaded with Mike, begging for an apology or anything, but he didn't say a word. He just watched Tim, almost as if he didn't recognize him. It had been almost twenty years since he killed himself. Tim took a step back and just watched his brother.

Mike stayed there for a minute, just watching Tim, never saying a word; his face didn't show sadness or anger...just acceptance before he too was gone.

"Mike! Come back, please!"

Tim had always felt like there was so much more to say to Mike—so many apologies for not being there for him when he needed it, for not being a better brother, and for not being with him in those final moments. He had always wondered if there was anything he could have done to stop it. Maybe he could have talked Mike out of picking up that rope. Maybe he could have done something—anything—because being able to try was better than how he found his brother...lifeless and alone.

But when the time came to speak, Tim felt frozen. He couldn't formulate the words he wanted to, and nothing came out.

"Fuck!" he screamed, standing up and punching the wall in front of him.

"You've not changed; you have to solve every problem with your fists."

"No, no, no, please, not you! I can't do this!" Tim closed his eyes and dropped to his knees, covering his head with his arms and cowering.

"I'm not leaving," she said, moving around the room.

Tim fought himself to look up; he couldn't bring himself to do it. He knew how much it would hurt.

She moved closer, knelt, and ran her hand along his back.

He raised his head, and there she was—those brown eyes, those brown eyes that had held his heart since the day he first saw her. The same soft, sweet smile that sent butterflies through his chest.

"You gonna apologize to me?" she chuckled.

"I let you down," he said, the tears that had trickled now running violently down his face.

"Oh, you poor baby!" She moved a little closer to Tim and ran her hand along his cheek. He could feel the warmth of her fingers— that touch he had thought about for so long, something he thought he would never see again.

"You never let me down," she said, looking deep into his eyes as he wept, trying so hard to stop himself, but to no avail.

Tim sniffled, attempting to regain his composure as he pulled himself to his feet.

"What?" he asked.

Hannah stood to meet his gaze, still smiling. She followed him, her eyes matching his. She ran her hand up his arm before pulling him close.

"T, you knew you could never let me down," she said, tilting her head and trying to get a better look at him.

"But Sam?"

"You were protecting me. I never blamed you for that! I blamed myself; that was my fault! I should have listened to you."

"I must be hallucinating because you've never admitted you were wrong before," Tim chuckled.

Hannah moved closer to Tim, wrapping her soft hands around his head and pulling him down to kiss his forehead. He could feel her lips pressed against him as she ran her fingers through his black and grey hair and pulled him in.

The smell of peonies and carnations filled the air. Tim never forgot the scent of her favorite perfume; after she left, he would spray his pillow with it now and again just to remember her presence, just to feel that comfort he lost when she left.

"So, why did you leave?" he asked gently.

"T," she said, pulling her forehead to his, holding him closely, both their eyes closed.

And like that, she was gone.

Tim had spent so long feeling broken, ashamed, and alone in a world that seemed hell-bent on destroying whatever fragments of his soul remained. But in this moment, he hadn't found peace; he knew for the first time in a long time that it was possible.

CHAPTER 14

"I believe that what we become depends on what our fathers teach us at odd moments when they aren't trying to teach us. We are formed by little scraps of wisdom."

- **Umberto Eco** -

Luke had always had a way of just getting by without letting much faze him. Every time Norm had asked about his mum, he would just smile and reply, "It is what it is!"

Making his way through town today had been a rush for him. He thrived on the high stress and the heavy traffic; slowing down was where he sank.

"Excuse me," he said loudly, walking into the weirdly placed suit shop that sat between two tanning salons and across from one of the many pastry shops in Wakefield.

The tall woman who worked there raised her nose from across the store before walking towards him slowly.

"What do you want?" she asked, emphasizing the first syllable of each word.

"I want to sell suits," he replied, smiling.

"Do you have suit-selling experience?" she asked, still looking at him from the edge of her nose.

"Nope, how do I get that?" he asked, reveling in the frustration he could see building in her face.

"You need to sell suits."

"Great! So can I get a job?" he asked, her head nearly exploding at this point.

The woman didn't say another word; she huffed and turned away from Luke before storming to the back of the shop, refusing to look back.

He watched her closely, and as soon as she moved out of sight, he grabbed the nice low tops he had seen through the window and made his way back out, disappearing into the busy crowd.

Luke bobbed and weaved through the crowd, slipping effortlessly through, rarely stopping for much except maybe the odd wallet or left phone.

"Excuse me, miss," he shouted, noticing a young lady in a long green dress had dropped her purse out of her back pocket. She turned to look at him, saw the ragged shoes he had been wearing and the tattered backpack, then turned straight around and walked off, ignoring anything else he would have to say.

"Yoink!" Luke chuckled to himself, slipping the purse into his bag.

He made his way back home, slipping into the hotel and ducking past the reception desk, straight up to Tim's room. As he moved closer, he could hear Tim shouting to himself, so he stopped and just listened.

He slowly crept open the door and watched Tim, pale and sweating profusely; he couldn't leave. Dad wouldn't. He watched as Tim fell to his knees, muttering "Hannah" under his breath before falling unconscious.

Luke moved around the hotel room quickly, trying to prop up Tim's head and wrap him in whatever he could find. He wasn't sure what was wrong, but he knew enough—his skin was cold, and he had fallen at some point, as blood trickled from his nose and a small gash appeared at the top of his head.

Luke sat with Tim all night, not leaving his side except to grab water and change the towels he had sweated through.

"Hannah," he muttered, a quiet despair in his voice.

The hallucinations intensified as Tim slipped in and out of consciousness; at one point, he felt like everyone he had ever wronged or pissed off had passed by. He felt like he was wrestling his brain for control. The pain and torment twisted his mind as he writhed in agony. Was this it? He thought to himself. Was this how it ended? No battle or war, no final fight—just cold sweats and fever.

Through his blurred vision, he looked out into the room ahead, his face down, beads of sweat running down his head. He saw her one last time. She didn't say anything this time; she just walked towards him, crouched down beside him, and ran her soft hands through his hair. He could see the sparkle in her brown eyes and the star-shaped necklace he had bought her years ago, the one she loved at first sight but couldn't bring herself to buy.

There wasn't a part of her that he hadn't fallen in love with—from her soft cheeks and big smile to the lines under her eyes she always complained about. He would kiss every single centimeter of her if she would let him.

And that smile, the one she only had for him. Nothing in the world mattered if he knew he could get home to that smile.

It was her. In every lifetime, it was always her. As she crouched down, her hair fell across her face; she had always complained it was too long, but they both knew if she ever cut it, her heart would break. He loved it; he was enamored by every single one of these things.

He had put it down to a combination of things. Tim's youth had been vicious; his first memories were of violence and loneliness. He remembered waking up one night to the sounds of smashing, sirens, and screaming. He couldn't have been any older than four years old. He remembered following the noise, but everything was so dark in the house.

Before he knew it, the entire house was quiet. He crept into the pitch-black living room; everything was dark except for the static from the TV. Then he saw it in the darkness: his father sat there, bottle in hand, almost invisible, the light reflecting off his blood-red eyes. Tim thought it was the devil.

His father just watched Tim, pure hatred in his eyes, whiskey dripping off his top lip. He lit a cigarette before ushering Tim towards him. He wasn't sure what had happened, but he knew in the commotion everyone had left him behind; it wouldn't be the last time.

And for the first time in his life, Tim knew real fear. Tim had known nothing but violence and loneliness his entire life; he had become a student of war. He was a protector, and at one point in his life, there wasn't anything he wouldn't do if it meant protecting his brothers. There wasn't a thing too far for him.

Then he met her. There she came, grey jumper, double-strapped backpack, and a big smile. That was it; for the first time in his life, he got to experience real beauty. More than that, he got to experience a love and purity he had never thought possible. He fought himself every single day because how could he deserve this?

Tim fell for Hannah because, for the first time in his life, he saw that there was a life beyond the battlefield. And there she was, looking into his eyes without saying a word.

"I can't do this anymore," he cried.

When he had passed out back in the flat, he felt nothing. She was safe, and that was all that mattered. He could hear the beeping from the monitors the EMTs had wheeled in; he could hear his lifeline. The doctors around him discussed whether he would make it to the hospital or not.

And then it was time to let go. He knew it; he could feel his heart rate slowing. He was drifting. There wasn't much time. He tried to open his eyes to take one final look at Hannah, but they wouldn't work. He could feel her hand in his; he tried to ball a fist, to squeeze her and maybe let her know he was okay, but his hands wouldn't work.

It was time to let go. It's important to know when the fights are over. But then Hannah did it.

"Please don't leave me," she begged. He could feel her desperation, how hard she squeezed his hands. He could hear the paramedics trying to console her.

And like that, the next battle started.

"I would have died for you a thousand times in a thousand lifetimes," he would always tell her... Now it was time to live for her.

CHAPTER 15

"Never lose hope. Storms make people stronger and never last forever."
- Roy T. Bennett -

As the night wore on, Tim could feel his fever dissipate. He knew it would never be that easy, over like that, but slowly it died away. She stayed, though.

Why did she stay?

"What are you trying to tell me?" he would ask between bouts of blurred vision and shakes that he thought would rattle his teeth from his mouth. But she didn't say a word; she just stayed with him and comforted him. She would hold his arm the same way she used to run her fingers through his hair and smile when her fingers reached the gray patches.

"Who's Hannah?" Luke asked, watching Tim slowly fall out of his hysteria.

"She's the love of my life."

"Where is she?"

"Gone."

And that was that. Luke knew enough; he didn't ask again.

"Here, that'll make you feel better," Luke said, pulling out one of the purses he had taken earlier that day. "This lady—posh, very snooty," he chuckled. "Carries a George

Clooney Batman trading card." He laughed, noticing Tim's facial expression remaining almost perplexed. "Maybe you had to see how posh this lady was... Either way, I'm keeping this," he said, slipping the card into his front pocket.

"Thank you," Tim said, smiling.

He never handled positivity too well; he found it hard to trust. It's a difficult transition when you are raised in a home like Tim's; it can be very hard to believe anyone can be nice for the sake of being nice. Sometimes it takes a minute.

But Tim trusted Luke and Norman. There was something about them that made him know they were good people.

That night, Luke barely left Tim's side. He watched him writhe and tried his best to keep him calm when he could, but they both knew Tim had to ride this out.

"When this dies down, I think you should come home," Luke suggested.

They had decided between them that this was the best option. Luke wrapped Tim up, and they made their way out into the cold night air.

Luke almost carried Tim through the house, leading him upstairs and dropping him into the spare bedroom. He wrapped him up and left him, heading off to sleep.

"Shout if you need me," he said before turning around and heading out.

She had followed.

Still not a word.

Tim pulled himself off the bed and onto the floor, dragging the duvet with him. He looked into her eyes, closed them, and pulled her forehead towards his, feeling her warmth one last time.

And like that... she was gone.

Tim awoke in the early hours of the next morning to the sounds of smashing. Pulling himself to his wobbling feet, he ran across the landing, following the noise. He burst into Luke's room and stood there, broken glass around him, clutching a brick.

"Someone threw this," he said, worry in his voice.

Tim moved over the broken glass, looked through the now-smashed window, and stood there on the beach. The young lad hadn't even thought about seeing him the day before.

But he wasn't alone. Standing next to him was a handful of men dressed in black. They looked at Tim for what felt like an hour, just staring back and forth before they scattered.

"What are we going to do?" Luke asked, stepping over the broken pieces and making his way to Tim.

"Nothing. Grab a brush; I'll clean this up and fix the window. They aren't worth the stress."

And that's what he did. Tim got stuck in, boarded up the window, and had it replaced in a day. His focus couldn't be pulled away from his recovery; he knew that. He knew he was in no state or shape to fight.

But Tim could stay busy. He could fix the house, repair what needed to be repaired. He figured now that they had gotten their revenge, that would be it. They would go away, stroke each other's egos, and tell each other how tough they were.

The following few days were quiet. Tim found himself staying there, and the longer he stayed, the more they bonded. Tim and Norm would swap war stories, and Norm had come to appreciate the company.

For Luke, it was like having a big brother—albeit a cool one who smoked and punched people. "All he needs is a leather jacket," he would joke.

CHAPTER 16

"The loneliest moment in someone's life is when they are watching their whole world fall apart, and all they can do is stare blankly."

- F. Scott Fitzgerald -

Tim sat alone, his bare feet pressed into the beach sand as he watched the sunset over the water. There had always been comfort in solitude for Tim. He loved people, but he enjoyed watching from the outside—like being outside of a party, enjoying a smoke, listening to the music, and savoring those small moments of tranquility.

He felt the cigarette smoke filling his lungs as he listened to the waves crash gently.

"The first time I came and sat here, you held my arm; do you remember?" Tim whispered to Hannah. He knew she wasn't there, but with her being his last hallucination—one that refused to go—he found himself thinking.

"You've got to let me go," he said as she moved across and wrapped both her arms around his before resting her head on his shoulder.

"I think I get it now... you never blamed me, did you?"

She tilted her head up to look at him.

"You blamed yourself."

She squeezed his arm a little tighter before kissing him on the cheek.

"Are you still seeing her?" Luke asked, walking up and sitting beside Tim.

"I am."

Most people talk about fight or flight when it comes to trauma response, but there are five different responses: freeze, flop, and fawn are the less talked about. From the outside of the situation, it's easy to miss a lot of these nuances, just as we often don't have time to process the consequences these actions can have on the world around us.

A wise man once said we are all, all of us, a different person to someone. Some people will see you as empathetic; some, hostile. It is during these moments we learn who we are.

Tim froze the first time he saw his dad become violent. He had always worried that he fawned for Hannah. He tried not to burden her or put too much pressure on her, and it took a long time for him to open up. There's no way to describe the feeling of opening up those wounds for someone only for them to leave.

Like all wounds, they can make or break us; they define our futures, our actions, and how we treat people. It's easy to forget as we go through life, day by day. The easiest thing you can do is let those wounds be the reason you affect someone else... it's how you affect them that matters.

At fifteen, Tim's actions were those of violence. He shouldered the burdens of the world and became the shield to his brothers, the sword when they needed it, so they didn't have to. But our actions always have consequences.

"Let's go!" Tim shouted. At fifteen years old, he had set off with his brothers and a friend, Harry, to make a little cash. Another weekend, another rave.

These things always went down the same: Mike would stick with Tim, and they would sell whatever they could, usually sugar water they passed off as a drug enhancer. Eddie would stick a little further behind for backup, and Harry would hold the money. Although the money was good, they reveled in making the rich kids look a little stupid and took whatever opportunity they could to stash a little loot, whether that be wallets or jewelry. If it could be lifted, it could be sold.

This time was no different from any other. The usual crowd gathered: young girls sipping vodka straight from the bottle and showing off whatever they had brought with daddy's money. The lads were just as predictable, with tight shirts, body odor, and cheap aftershave.

The boys generally skirted by on reputation, but being the only ones there not born with a silver spoon, they came across a little rougher than the rest.

"Here you go, love," Tim shouted, music blaring, slipping somebody a vial of sugar water. With every single sale, he would give Mike a nudge.

"Fucking idiots," he laughed.

As the night wore on, Harry became very aware of the amount of money he now held, slipping three hundred plus pounds into his inside coat. His eyes shifted, sensing that someone was watching him.

"We need to go!" he shouted, trying to get Mike's attention, but Mike brushed him off and carried on. The boys didn't care; the music was good, and the money was stacking up. Why would they leave so early?

As more people piled in, Harry tightened his coat, becoming more paranoid by the second as he watched the crowd disappear around Tim and Mike.

"Fuck," he thought to himself as he looked back—Eddie was gone too. He took a second to decide to make his way to the exit. As he turned back, the eyes had now fixed on him.

He turned again and moved through the crowd, watching over his shoulder. He could see that they were now making a beeline for him.

He picked up the pace and barged his way through the crowd, knocking over whoever got in his way. Every path he tried to take seemed to be blocked, and before he knew it, he was surrounded.

Turning around, he saw a man in a white shirt and blue jeans, his shirt unbuttoned down to the bottom of his chest and with more hair gel than any one man should ever use. Harry watched as the man reached out to try and grab him.

He slipped past him and started running for the exit, not looking back to see if they had continued chasing him. As he slipped out into the cold night air, he felt something knock the wind out of him as he fell to his feet.

He turned around, and there he stood. Under better circumstances, he'd have taken the mick out of the shirt-and-blue-jeans combo, but in this moment, as fear set in, all he could think of was getting out of there.

He tried to pick himself up, but when he put a hand down to lift himself, he felt another knock, this time on his head, then another. Before he knew it, he was being kicked from all directions.

"How many are there?" he thought in desperate panic as he rolled onto his front and covered his head. The noise was so loud that he hadn't noticed the crowd that had formed around him; none of them did anything—they just watched, frozen.

"Eddie!" he screamed, seeing his friend through the blur of blood running down his face. The man in white turned and looked at Eddie, but he didn't say a word; he just looked on blankly, putting his hands up and trying to reason with the men.

Tim burst through the crowd and, in an instant, had turned the man's white shirt red, sending him hurtling to the floor and cracking his head on the pavement. The man tried to steady himself and sit up.

"Cunt!" Tim shouted, immediately following up with a boot to the face, taking him out of the fight quicker than his brain had time to process.

"You've sold us fucking duds!" one of the group shouted, moving towards Tim, his chest puffed out, trying to come across as somewhat intimidating. Without much thought, Tim threw a headbutt that put him down as well, and before he knew it, Mike was there.

And that was it.

Anarchy.

The venue descended into chaos as every man started throwing punches. Most didn't even know why or who they were hitting, but it didn't matter to the boys; they had been messed with, and it was more important to send a message.

Harry watched in horror as the bodies piled around him, people falling to their feet, trying to escape. He could hear screaming and thudding as he pulled himself up, his head spinning. Through blurred vision, he pushed his way through, trying to get to a safe distance.

He pushed and pushed, trying with everything he had to get out. He felt his lungs tighten; every ounce of strength he had felt like it had been ripped from his body.

As he made his way to a clearing, he ran over the road and threw himself down onto a patch of grass. He looked on in horror at the sight ahead of him. How had it escalated so quickly over a little bit of money and a man's ego?

Harry fought desperately, trying to regain his breath; the fear and anxiety had ripped through his chest, taking everything he had. As he fought to regain some sense of self-control, he looked up, and there he was—the now red-shirted fool who had started this.

"No, please, we don't need to do this," he pleaded.

Tim had tried to follow Harry, and as he pushed his way through the crowd, forcing people out of the way, he broke through to a clearing. In the distance, he saw Harry, who had put his hands up. Through blurred sight and a struggle to breathe, he pleaded desperately, "I don't want to fight you. Here, you can have the money." As he reached into his pocket, he realized he was past money at this point. This was about pride and a broken, fragile ego.

The man threw a single punch at Harry, his eyes rolling back instantly. He was dead before he hit the ground.

There wasn't a single day for the rest of Tim's life that he didn't blame himself for that. Mike, too; Eddie would never bring himself to tell Tim that he could have stopped it that night.

After that night, a lot of things changed for Tim. He became more violent, more unrelenting; he was never going to let that happen again, and he would go as far as he needed to ensure that he and the ones closest to him made it home. He had always been the one to carry the burden of violence, to do the things that needed to be done to make sure the boys got home safely, to make sure they ate and stayed as safe as they could be in this life.

Until he met Hannah.

He didn't need to be that person with her; she had shown him there was another way, that it was okay to take a step back before responding.

And despite everything, despite all of the things he had done, he was worthy of love—something he thought was lost on someone like him.

CHAPTER 17

*D*ear Hannah,
    I'm still alive, who'd have thought it?
I've met some people, good people.
They need me here,
although I think I need them more.
I need to let you go.
I will love you until the end of time,
until I run out of breath,
in this life and whatever comes next.
But I have to let you go.
I love you this much.
Goodbye, Han.
T.

CHAPTER 18

Tim wrote the final letter he would pen on this journey, folding it and putting it away. He may never send this one, but for his peace of mind, it felt good to write.

That night, they all sat together, watching the sun go down over the beach from the front decking, country music playing quietly.

"You're a good man, Tim," Norm smiled, relaxing back in his chair. He pulled his flat cap down over his head and drifted off.

Tim would never admit it, but as those words left Norm's mouth, he bit his lip hard, trying to stop himself from welling up. Maybe it was the withdrawal that made him emotional; either way, he didn't like it. He appreciated it, though. He would never get the chance to tell Norm how much his kindness meant to him, but Norm knew. Sometimes in life, some things don't need to be said. Norm was from a different time, a time when not everything needed to be spelled out and made clear verbally. It's a person's actions you should judge, he had always thought.

As Norm drifted off, Tim picked him up and carried him to his bed before making his way back out onto the front deck. Something about this view made him feel at peace.

"Here," Luke said quietly, handing him a cola and sitting down next to him. They didn't say another word.

Tim had hoped getting to this point would end the hallucinations. He loved Hannah more than he could put down on paper, but seeing her in the manner he was had broken him. But there she stayed—silent still.

Making his way through town, Tim took a slower path than usual. He stopped to appreciate the weather a little more, to watch the people racing by. He hadn't planned to make it this far. Now that he was here, he felt a little more grateful for the little things.

Still unsure of what the future would hold, all he knew was that he wasn't finished here. Market squares in Wakefield weren't much different from anywhere else—families selling out of their cars, stalls filled with useless junk, and old VHS tapes he chuckled at while walking past.

Looking up through the crowd, Tim saw a face he recognized all too well—the man who had attacked him. Maybe he could get some revenge for throwing the brick. Tim looked around for Luke, who had a bad habit of showing up at the worst times, but there was no sign of him. He began making his way toward his attacker.

Before he could reach him, Hannah appeared, stopping Tim in his tracks and placing a hand on his chest. He just looked into her eyes; she didn't need to say anything.

Tim turned to walk away, but he was stopped by another figure—this one bigger than the first—who moved quickly toward him, almost knocking down the poor shoppers who had just been browsing. Knowing he had to leave, Tim slipped to the right and disappeared through the back of a clothing shop.

He knew this wasn't over, but maybe there was a way to end it without more bloodshed. Before leaving for Wakefield, Tim had sold everything—his flat and almost everything he owned. He had one final beer with his brothers and sat with Eddie at Mike's grave, sharing a last drink together. Eddie was unaware of any ill intentions Tim had; nonetheless, he savored the moment.

Tim had covered almost every base; everything was set. In the three weeks he had stayed in Wakefield, everything had changed. With Norm and Luke, he had found the family he had never really had. He might not have found peace, but he was closer than he had ever thought he would get.

All the things in life he had dreamed of—a wife, kids, a real family, big Saturday BBQs, and pancakes on Sundays—seemed so distant now. He had envisioned all the ways he would make Hannah feel loved and appreciated: running her a nice bath after a long day, bringing her breakfast in bed, and finding cheap crisps she always loved. He had dreamed of creating the family he never had.

Sitting outside the house he grew up in at eight years old, scared to go inside, had cemented in his mind that his kids would never go through what he did—what his brothers did. All of those dreams died when Hannah left. He had to come to terms not only with the end of their relationship but also with the death of the future they had both planned.

That's the thing about heartbreak people don't speak about: you aren't just losing the person; you're losing the life you both started building together. The destination you set out for is gone, and now the road behind you has cracked. In the beginning, that heartache was almost paralyzing.

Some people never get back up from that feeling; some wear it like armor, never letting anyone in again, and then some use that pain to heal those who need it. Pain is funny that way: you can use it as an excuse to screw the world, destroy everything in your path, or you can use it to pave the road ahead.

During the first argument Tim had with Hannah, he stormed out. He meant no malice; it was more to give them both time to calm down and let saner heads prevail. When he came back, she was silent, watching the sunset through her bedroom window, tears welling in her eyes. She had thought that he left her, but he decided then and there that no matter the issue, no matter how big or small, he wouldn't leave until he knew things were fixed. He would hold her all night if he needed to—anything to reassure her that he wasn't going anywhere.

He would wake every morning now the same way. He would roll over to check on her, wrap his arms around her, and the stark realization that she was gone and wasn't coming home would set in. And like that, he was up. It didn't matter the time of day or night; that's all it would take for him not to get back to sleep, no matter what he did.

He would roll out of bed, sleep deprivation or not, and he would make his bed—always the first mission of the day. This day was no different from any other. He awoke in the early hours of the morning, rolling over; his hand landed on the space in the bed across from him. Even in his hallucinated state, Hannah wouldn't be there in bed with him. He pulled his tired body to his feet and made his bed.

Tim stared blankly into his bathroom mirror, looking at the large scars that ran along his abdomen, back, and arms—all marked with their own stories. Some were admittedly more traumatic than others: the scarring on his thumb was from when his dad had given it to him once for putting his hands up, refusing to fight him. His dad had latched onto his thumb with his teeth and gnawed down; then there were the six stitches on his leg from trying to make Hannah laugh with his dancing and ending up falling into a wishing well—some irony there.

He made his way downstairs to have breakfast with Luke and Norm, and like most mornings, Norm would moan about the state of the world while reading the daily paper before they would both mock him over coffee. Tim had set out to fix the front garden; he had worked tirelessly with Norm's input, trying to get it somewhere in the region of where it used to be. He would help Luke with his homework, maybe try to get him to help out with some of the physical labor. Above everything, he was just trying to be better than the day before.

As the day wore on, Tim watched the sun go down from the front garden. He admired the orange vista that encapsulated the entire sky as it turned an almost fire red. He felt the cold breeze rushing over his face, and looking up at the front decking, he could see the two just laughing. Tim pulled out the last letter he wrote and made his way out of the front garden; it was time to post it.

Time to say goodbye.

"I hope you are getting these," he said to the hallucinatory Hannah, who had watched him post the letter with a look of sadness and understanding in her eyes before he made his way back to the house. Norm greeted him as he walked back up before ushering Luke inside.

"You know that boy thinks the world of you, you know," Norm said with a wry smile.

"He's a good kid."

"Well, you're not bad yourself—pretty damn good with some shears as well. We were wondering if you wanted to stay here with us. We know you haven't been here long, but you're family. You don't have to answer yet, but I want you to know we both appreciate you, and we'll respect any decision you make... as long as you still do a little gardening for us." He chuckled, slipping a wink at Tim.

CHAPTER 19

If you want peace,
Prepare for war.
- Latin Proverb -

Tim awoke that night the same as every other, rolling over to wrap his arms around Hannah. As he rolled over that night, there she lay, staring back at him, those brown eyes lighting up the dark room. He ran his hand along the space, took a deep breath, and pulled himself up.

The house was silent, not a noise inside or out. He just lay there for a moment, waiting for the realization that she wasn't there, that feeling of dread filling his chest. When he heard a smash, it was louder than the last time; this wasn't a brick. He jumped up and made his way for the door, running into Luke's room to see Luke panicked.

"In your dad's room now!"

Before making his way back out and down the creaking stairs, he could see broken glass covering the floor. The front door had been smashed open, knocking debris everywhere and covering the floor.

"Don't come down here!" he shouted back up, running out the front door to look for any signs of those who did this. There was nothing. The night was silent.

He turned to make his way back into the house. In the kitchen, he grabbed a rolling pin—the first thing he found that he thought could be used as a weapon. Turning back into the living room, it was as if a hurricane had passed through.

Suddenly, he felt a crack across his back, sending him hurtling to the floor. Before he had time to process what was going on, he felt another smash, this time across his head, knocking him completely out.

He awoke to the sounds of arguing and screaming. Everything was a blur, and his head spun as he struggled to see through the blood pouring down his forehead.

"Tim, please wake up," he knew that voice.

"Tim!"

He watched in horror as he saw them—the men. They had pulled Luke and Norman downstairs. Luke had blood smeared across his face, but it was almost impossible to tell where it had come from. The only areas of Tim's face he could see were the tracks of tears that had run down his cheeks.

"We were just meant to scare them! Now look what you've done, dickhead!"

As Tim pulled himself out of his daze, he could see them—three of them arguing among themselves, as one tried to block the front door to stop any passersby from seeing what they had done. Through bloodied vision, he scanned the room. One more held Luke, slapping him every time he tried to wriggle out of his grip, and one more behind Tim had pulled him to his knees and hadn't said a word as the rest argued.

Between the three arguing men, a figure lay on the floor, blood pouring profusely from his head.

"We have to kill the rest right fucking now! Otherwise, we're all going to prison!" one of the voices screamed, looking down and kicking the body that lay by his feet.

Hannah crouched through, knelt in front of Tim, and raised a hand onto his chest. He scanned the room; he could see the fear in Luke's eyes. He could hear Norm gargling, convulsing on the floor as blood spat from his mouth.

"You know what I need to do," he said to Hannah, tears streaming down his face. "I've already lost you; I can't lose them as well!"

She looked at Tim with a pained smile, pulled her hand away, and stepped to the side.

"This guy's crazy!" one of the voices shouted, seeing Tim wrestling with his own mind.

The escalation of violence has been a constant throughout human history; wars have been waged due to pride and egos. This was no different; sometimes all it takes is a look, a funny turn, or a misunderstanding.

More men have died due to pride than any other cause. And like that, she was gone. Tim threw his head back hard, smashing the nose of the man behind him and instantly splitting it in two. He jumped to his feet, turned, and ripped the bat from his hands before smashing it as hard as he could into his forehead.

The man fell to the floor, clutching at the bone protruding from his nose and spluttering blood into the air, gasping for breath. Tim raised his foot and smashed down as hard as he could onto his knee, shattering it instantly. He stomped and stomped, sending blood spraying up the walls until he heard footsteps coming from behind.

He turned to see one of the men running for him. With both hands, he swung the bat at the man's face, missing and hitting his windpipe; that was two out. In the carnage, Luke had immediately run for Norman and pulled him out of the way into the adjoining room, keeping his head low.

Tim stood there, clutching the bat as the three men stood in front of him, hesitant to make a move. They knew he wasn't going down without a fight, and he was ready. He wasn't going to let anyone else suffer because of him... well, that wasn't a hundred percent true.

One of the men stepped forward, and Tim swung the bat, almost taking himself off his feet. As another grabbed him from behind and the instigator swung for him, he raised his arm and ricocheted the punch off his elbow, shattering the man's knuckles. He threw the bat again as it smashed in two on the side of one of the men. Seeing it had broken and splintered, he immediately drove the sharp, jagged edge straight into the man's chest, sending him flat on his back and screaming in pain. He clutched the bat handle sticking out of his chest, coughing blood as his eyes streamed with tears. Between the carnage, all the noise, and destruction, Luke swore he could hear him begging for his mum.

The man who had grabbed Tim from behind began cracking him with punches, desperately trying to throw anything he had at Tim. Tim pulled at the man's arm, raised it over his shoulder, and pulled down hard, cracking his arm in two.

He turned, still holding the arm, and grabbed the man from the back of the head before driving it into the wall behind him, breaking his nose. He pulled his head back and slammed it again repeatedly, the sound of shattering bones becoming louder with each impact until the man had become unrecognizable.

"Tim!" Luke screamed. As he turned around, he could see the final man grabbing Luke and pulling him in front of him.

"Let me go, or I'll kill him! Do not fucking test me!"

Tim, still holding the guy's now bloodied head, dropped him, sending him crashing straight to the floor. He looked around at the blood pooled on the floor, the broken furniture, and the now red walls. The men lay about the floor, clutching their broken parts, some worse for wear than others. Tim was covered, head to toe, in sprayed blood and fragments of human flesh that he couldn't identify if you'd asked him. He breathed heavily, adrenaline pumping through him, and looked Luke dead in the eyes.

Luke looked back at him and just nodded. Tim made his way to the man.

"Don't you fucking dare!"

Luke dropped to the floor and rolled out of the way, running to grab his dad. He tried his best to drag him to safety, but knowing he wasn't strong enough, he did what he could to stem the bleeding.

"Stay with me, please, Dad," he begged, holding tightly. He could feel Norm's hand squeezing his as he struggled to breathe, his eyes bloodshot as they darted around the room.

"I'm right here," he cried.

Norm squeezed Luke's hand tightly, looked into his eyes, and smiled as his hands went cold and the squeeze became softer.

"Please, Dad!" Luke put his head to his father's chest, listening to his breathing slowly, and like that... the beating stopped.

Running at the man as he tried to backtrack, Tim grabbed him and threw him to the floor, stomping on his already broken hand. Using his other hand, he reached into the burnt-out fireplace and grabbed a handful of whatever he could, throwing it into the man's eyes, blinding him temporarily.

The man picked up the fire poker that sat next to the fireplace and began swinging it at Tim. The first swing broke his forearm. Swinging repeatedly out of desperation, he hit Tim again, and as he went to swing again, Luke lunged at the man, knocking him off his feet.

He stood immediately and cracked Luke once with the fire poker, sending blood spraying up the walls as Luke crashed to the floor.

Tim pulled himself to his feet, ran at the man, and smashed his head into his nose hard before pulling back and ripping at his throat with his teeth. Pulling a chunk of windpipe out, he watched as the man took a step back, clutched at his throat, and then took a single gurgle before falling back, crashing into the floor.

Tim ran for Luke and rolled him over, seeing the bruising on his face; his eye had swollen almost immediately.

"Did we win?"

Tim helped Luke to his feet as they rushed to Norman. He was gone.

The following days passed by in a blur. Between police interviews and hospital trips, they hadn't had time to process the events of that night. Luke stayed by Tim's side as they restructured his arm.

The police explained that the attackers had been going house to house for months; they weren't the first to be attacked.

But they would be the last.

CHAPTER 20

Dear Dad,
I kept your flat cap.

I hope you don't mind. I'm sorry I couldn't protect you. I know Tim is as well.

You taught me what it is to be a man, and you showed me the value of respect and kindness, even when the world didn't show you.

I promise I'll make you proud.

We buried you today, just me and Tim.

Mum came back today, she came for the house, she can have it, she doesn't get me.

I found a brother in Tim.

I'm going to go and stay with him, he needs me, more than he'll ever admit.

I'll see you again.

Luke.

CHAPTER 21

"You ready, bud?" Tim had said to Luke, creaking open the door to his bedroom.

"Yes, sir," he said excitedly, jumping up and grabbing his school bag. Tim had rented a flat not five minutes from Norman's old house. It hadn't been an easy few months; between everything that had happened and adjusting to life after trauma, it affects everyone differently.

Luke had struggled, blaming himself. He lost more than a father that day; he lost his best friend and his home. But he found a brother in Tim and trusted him when he said everything was going to be okay.

Oftentimes, it can be hard to adjust back to reality after such events. It's important to count the little things, the ones closest to you. It's important to honor the past but never be afraid of embracing the future.

Tim walked Luke down to the bus stop and sat with him a while while the world passed by around them.

"What are you going to do?" Luke asked.

"I guess I should probably look at getting a job..." he chuckled.

As the bus pulled in, Luke grabbed his bag and threw it over his shoulder. He stood, and just before he jumped on, he turned and hugged Tim, squeezing him tightly.

"I'll see you later," he smiled.

CHAPTER 22

"And I'll dream each night for some version of you that I might not have but I did not lose"
- Noah Kahan -

Tim sat alone on the beach, the same beach where not long ago he had thought about killing himself. He thought back to the first time he came here; Hannah had held his arm as they watched the sun come down over the water. They had lit a small fire pit and spent the night just laughing. He remembered seeing the light from the fire reflected in her eyes, how the moonlight shone down on them, and feeling his heart swell when he looked at her. Every beat of his heart was hers from the moment they had met.

Now, he sat here alone, heart split in two, watching the waves crash. He pulled his arm out of the sling that had wrapped around his neck and lit a cigarette, watching those same waves gently crash along the rocks. The passage of time had worn them down, but they stood strong. That's the thing about damage: as all wounds heal, the scars remain in all things.

He thought back to the first time coming here, when he was going to end everything. It wasn't that long ago; he was going to kill himself right on this spot. The waves crashed as the cool air rolled over the sea. He felt the sand under him and the smoke filling his lungs, reflecting on all those memories—everything that had broken him, everything that had led him here.

Now was his chance at being a better man than he had been. Tim closed his eyes and took a breath, soaking in all that was around him. He didn't know what the future would hold or how it would play out. But for the first time in a long time, he was hopeful.

Tim heard the crunching of sand and felt a hand on his shoulder. He spun around, preparing himself for trouble.

"Hey, T."

"Hannah..."

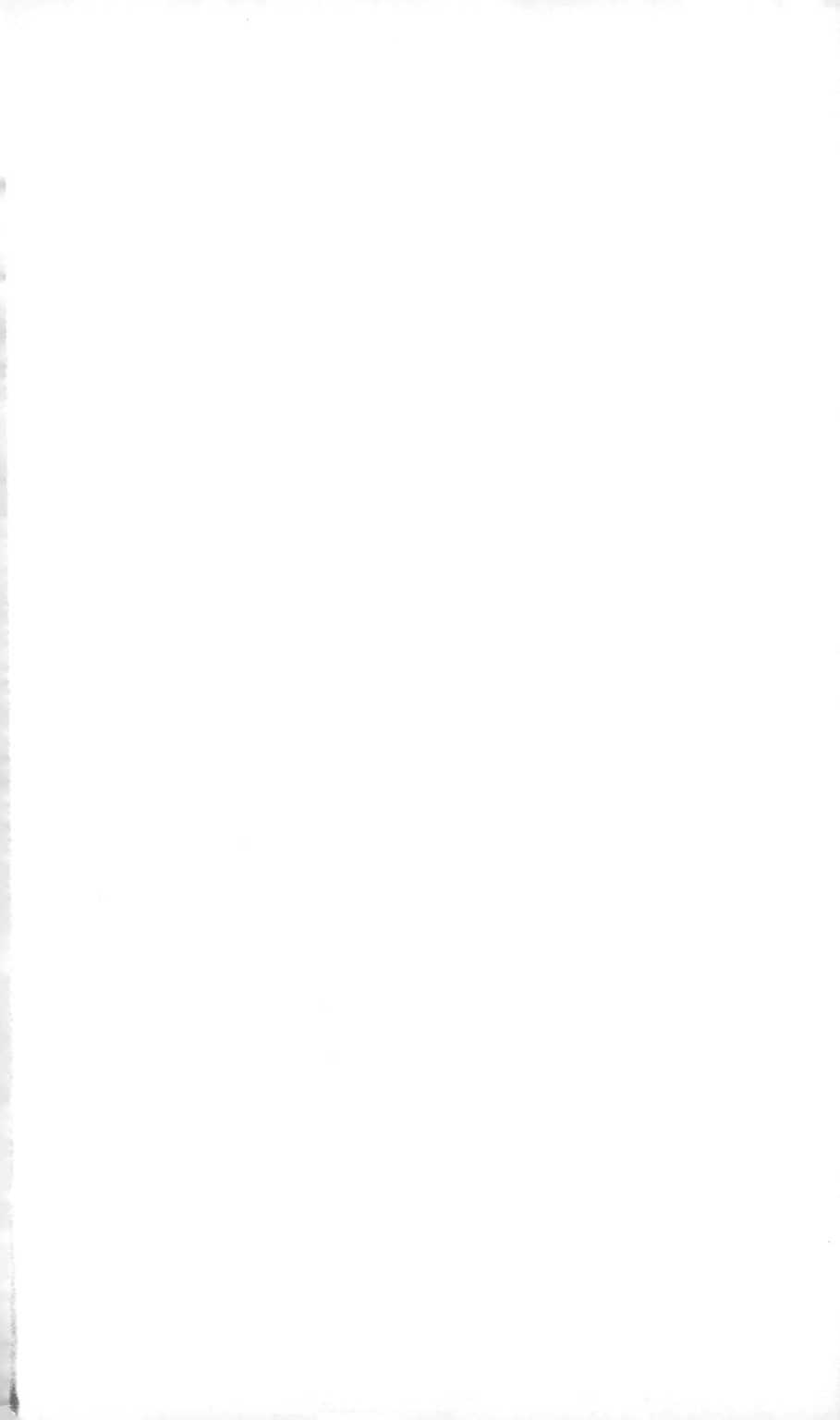

9 798896 863434